ADVANCES IN
HUMAN GENETICS 17

CONTRIBUTORS TO THIS VOLUME

Stylianos E. Antonarakis
Genetics Unit
Department of Pediatrics
The Johns Hopkins University School
 of Medicine
Baltimore, Maryland

Edwin A. Azen
Laboratory of Genetics and
Department of Medicine
University of Wisconsin
Madison, Wisconsin

Mitchell S. Golbus
Reproductive Genetics Unit
Department of Obstetrics and
 Gynecology
University of California, San
 Francisco
San Francisco, California

James D. Goldberg
Reproductive Genetics Unit
Department of Obstetrics and
 Gynecology
University of California, San
 Francisco
San Francisco, California

Terry J. Hassold
Division of Medical Genetics
Emory University
Atlanta, Georgia

Louis M. Kunkel
Division of Genetics and
 Mental Retardation Center
Children's Hospital and

Department of Pediatrics
Harvard Medical School and
Howard Hughes Medical Institute
Boston, Massachusetts and
Program in Neuroscience
Harvard University
Cambridge, Massachusetts

David M. Kurnit
University of Michigan Medical
 Center
Departments of Pediatrics and
 Human Genetics
Howard Hughes Medical Institute
Ann Arbor, Michigan

Nobuyo Maeda
Laboratory of Genetics
University of Wisconsin
Madison, Wisconsin

Anthony P. Monaco
Division of Genetics and
 Mental Retardation Center
Children's Hospital and
Department of Pediatrics
Harvard Medical School
Boston, Massachusetts and
Program in Neuroscience
Harvard University
Cambridge, Massachusetts

Gordon D. Stewart
University of Michigan Medical
 Center
Department of Pediatrics
Howard Hughes Medical Institute
Ann Arbor, Michigan

ADVANCES IN HUMAN GENETICS 1

Edited by

Harry Harris

Harnwell Professor of Human Genetics
University of Pennsylvania, Philadelphia

and

Kurt Hirschhorn

Herbert H. Lehman Professor and Chairman of Pediatrics
Mount Sinai School of Medicine of The City University of New York

PLENUM PRESS • NEW YORK AND LONDON

The Library of Congress catalogued the first volume of this title as follows:

Advances in human genetics. 1—
 New York, Plenum Press, 1970—
  (1) v. illus. 24-cm.
  Editors: V. 1—   H. Harris and K. Hirschhorn.
 1. Human genetics—Collected works. I. Harris, Harry, ed. II. Hirschhorn, Kurt, 1926—
joint ed.
QH431.A1A32   573.2'1   77-84583

ISBN-13: 978-1-4612-8279-2   e-ISBN-13: 978-1-4613-0987-1
DOI: 10.1007/978-1-4613-0987-1

© 1988 Plenum Press, New York
A Division of Plenum Publishing Corporation
233 Spring Street, New York, N.Y. 10013

Softcover reprint of the hardcover 1st edition 1988

ARTICLES PLANNED FOR FUTURE VOLUMES

Biochemical Defects in Immunodeficiency • *Rochelle Hirschhorn*
Neonatal Lethal Chondrodystrophies • *Jurgen Spranger and P. Maroteaux*
Advances in Prenatal Genetic Diagnosis • *John C. Hobbins and Maurice J. Mahoney*
Malformation Syndromes Caused by Single Gene Defects • *Judith G. Hall*
Genetics of Collagen and Its Disorders • *Darwin J. Prockop, Mon-Li Chu, and Anne Olsen*
Genetic Screening Using the Tay–Sachs Model • *Michael M. Kaback*
Huntington Disease • *James F. Gusella*
Genetics of Hormone Receptors and Their Abnormalities • *Jesse Roth and Simeon I. Taylor*
The Major Histocompatibility Complex and Disease Susceptibility • *Hugh O. McDevitt, John Bell, Paul Travers, and John Todd*
Genetic Defects of Growth Hormone Synthesis and Action • *John A. Phillips*
Overgrowth Syndromes • *M. Michael Cohen, Jr.*
Chromosome Instability Syndromes • *Maimon Cohen*
Genetics of Platelet Disorders • *James G. White*
Lacticacidemias • *Brian H. Robinson*
Genetics of Human Mitochondrial DNA • *Douglas C. Wallace*

CONTENTS OF EARLIER VOLUMES

VOLUME 1 (1970)
Analysis of Pedigree Data • *J. H. Edwards*
Autoradiography in Human Cytogenetics • *Orlando J. Miller*
Genetics of Immunoglobulins • *H. Hugh Fudenberg and Noel E. Warner*
Human Genetics of Membrane Transport with Emphasis on Amino Acids • *Charles R. Scriver and Peter Hechtman*
Genetics of Disorders of Intestinal Digestion and Absorption • *Jean Frézal and Jean Rey*

VOLUME 2 (1971)
Glucose-6-Phosphate Dehydrogenase • *Henry N. Kirkman*
Albinism • *Carl J. Witkop, Jr.*
Acatalasemia • *Hugo Aebi and Hedi Suter*
Chromosomes and Abortion • *D. H. Carr*
A Biochemical Genetic View of Human Cell Culture • *William J. Mellman*

VOLUME 3 (1972)
Prenatal Detection of Genetic Disorders • *Henry L. Nadler*
Ganglioside Storage Diseases • *John S. O'Brien*
Induced Chromosomal Aberrations in Man • *Arthur D. Bloom*
Linkage Analysis Using Somatic Cell Hybrids • *Frank H. Ruddle*
The Structure and Function of Chromatin • *David E. Comings*

VOLUME 4 (1973)

Genetic Screening • *Harvey L. Levy*
Human Population Structure • *Chris Cannings and L. Cavalli-Sforza*
Status and Prospects of Research in Hereditary Deafness • *Walter E. Nance and Freeman E. McConnell*
Congenital Adrenal Hyperplasia • *Maria I. New and Lenore S. Levine*
Cytogenetic Aspects of Human Male Meiosis • *Maj Hultén and J. Lindsten*

VOLUME 5 (1975)

The Chondrodystrophies • *David L. Rimoin*
New Techniques in the Study of Human Chromosomes: Methods and Applications • *Bernard Dutrillaux and Jerome Lejeune*
The Thalassemias: Models for Analysis of Quantitative Gene Control • *David Kabat and Robert D. Koler*
Spontaneous Mutation in Man • *Friedrich Vogel and Rüdiger Rathenberg*
Genetic Screening Legislation • *Philip Reilly*

VOLUME 6 (1976)

Vitamin-Responsive Inherited Metabolic Disorders • *Leon E. Rosenberg*
Inherited Deficiency of Hypoxanthine-Guanine Phosphoribosyltransferase in X-Linked Uric Aciduria • *J. Edwin Seegmiller*
Hereditary Hemolytic Anemia Due to Enzyme Defects of Glycolysis • *Sergio Piomelli and Laurence Corash*
Population Structure of the Åland Islands, Finland • *James H. Mielke, Peter L. Workman, Johan Fellman, and Aldur W. Eriksson*
Population Genetics and Health Care Delivery: The Quebec Experience • *Claude Laberge*

VOLUME 7 (1976)

Biochemical Genetics of Carbonic Anhydrase • *Richard E. Tashian and Nicholas D. Carter*
Human Behavior Genetics • *Barton Childs, Joan M. Finucci, Malcolm S. Preston, and Ann E. Pulver*
Mammalian X-Chromosome Inactivation • *Stanley M. Gartler and Robert J. Andina*
Genetics of the Complement System • *Chester A. Alper and Fred S. Rosen*
Selective Systems in Somatic Cell Genetics • *Ernest H. Y. Chu and Sandra S. Powell*

VOLUME 8 (1977)

Genetics and Etiology of Human Cancer • *Alfred G. Knudson, Jr.*
Population Genetics Theory in Relation to the Neutralist-Selectionist Controversy • *Warren J. Ewens*
The Human α-Amylases • *A. Donald Merritt and Robert C. Karn*
The Genetic Aspects of Facial Abnormalities • *Robert J. Gorlin and William S. Boggs*
Some Facts and Fancies Relating to Chromosome Structure in Man • *H. J. Evans*

VOLUME 9 (1979)

Chromosome and Neoplasia • *David G. Harnden and A. M. R. Taylor*

Terminological, Diagnostic, Nosological, and Anatomical–Developmental
  Aspects of Developmental Defects in Man • *John M. Opitz, Jürgen
  Herrmann, James C. Pettersen, Edward T. Bersu, and Sharon C.
  Colacino*
Human Alphafetoprotein 1956-1978 • *Matteo Adinolfi*
Genetic Mechanisms Contributing to the Expression of the Human
  Hemoglobin Loci • *William P. Winter, Samir M. Hanash, and Donald
  L. Rucknagel*
Genetic Aspects of Folate Metabolism • *Richard W. Erbe*

VOLUME 10 (1980)
Biochemistry and Genetics of the ABO, Lewis, and P Blood Group Systems •
  Winifred M. Watkins
HLA – A Central Immunological Agency of Man • *D. Bernard Amos and D. D.
  Kostyu*
Linkage Analysis in Man • *P. Michael Conneally and Marian L. Rivas*
Sister Chromatid Exchanges • *Samuel A. Latt, Rhona R. Schreck, Kenneth S.
  Loveday, Charlotte P. Dougherty, and Charles F. Shuler*
Genetic Disorders of Male Sexual Differentiation • *Kaye R. Fichman, Barbara
  R. Migeon, and Claude J. Migeon*

VOLUME 11 (1981)
The Pi Polymorphism: Genetic, Biochemical, and Clinical Aspects of Human
  α_1-Antitrypsin • *Magne K. Fagerhol and Diane Wilson Cox*
Segregation Analysis • *R. C. Elston*
Genetic, Metabolic, and Biochemical Aspects of the Porphyrias • *Shigeru Sassa
  and Attallah Kappas*
The Molecular Genetics of Thalassemia • *Stuart H. Orkin and David G. Nathan*
Advances in the Treatment of Inherited Metabolic Diseases • *Robert J. Desnick
  and Gregory A. Gravowski*

VOLUME 12 (1982)
Genetic Disorders of Collagen Metabolism • *David W. Hollister, Peter H.
  Beyers, and Karen A. Holbrook*
Advances in Genetics in Dermatology • *Howard P. Baden and Philip A. Hooker*
Haptoglobin: The Evolutionary Product of Duplication, Unequal Crossing Over,
  and Point Mutation • *Barbara H. Bowman and Alexander Kurosky*
Models of Human Genetic Disease in Domestic Animals • *D. F. Patterson,
  M. E. Haskins, and P. F. Jezyk*
Mapping the Human Genome, Cloned Genes, DNA Polymorphisms, and
  Inherited Disease • *Thomas B. Shows, Alan Y. Sakaguchi, and
  Susan L. Naylor*

VOLUME 13 (1983)
The Genetics of Blood Coagulation • *John B. Graham, Emily S. Barrow, Howard
  M. Reisner, and Cora-Jean S. Edgell*
Marker (X)-Linked Mental Retardation • *Gillian Turner and Patricia Jacobs*
Human Antibody Genes: Evolutionary and Molecular Genetic Perspectives • *Jay
  W. Ellison and Leroy E. Hood*
Mutations Affecting Trace Elements in Humans and Animals: A Genetic Approach
  to an Understanding of Trace Elements • *D. M. Danks and J. Camakaris*
Phenylketonuria and Its Variants • *Seymour Kaufman*

VOLUME 14 (1985)

Cytogenetics of Pregnancy Wastage • *Andre Boué, Alfred Gropp, and Joëlle Boué*

Mutation in Human Populations • *James F. Crow and Carter Denniston*

Genetic Mutations Affecting Human Lipoprotein Metabolism • *Vassilis I. Zannis and Jan L. Breslow*

Glucose-6-Phosphate Dehydrogenase • *L. Luzzatto and G. Battistuzzi*

Steroid Sulfatase Deficiency and the Genetics of the Short Arm of the Human X Chromosome • *Larry J. Shapiro*

VOLUME 15 (1986)

Chromosomal Abnormalities in Leukemia and Lymphoma: Clinical and Biological Significance • *Michelle M. Le Beau and Janet D. Rowley*

An Algorithm for Comparing Two-Dimensional Electrophoretic Gels, with Particular Reference to the Study of Mutation • *Michael M. Skolnick and James V. Neel*

The Human Argininosuccinate Synthetase Locus and Citrullinemia • *Arthur L. Beaudet, William E. O'Brian, Hans-Georg O. Bock, Svend O. Freytag, and Tsung-Sheng Su*

Molecular Genetics of the Human Histocompatibility Complex • *Charles Auffray and Jack L. Strominger*

Genetics of Human Alcohol and Aldehyde Dehydrogenases • *Moyra Smith*

VOLUME 16 (1987)

Genetics of Lactose Digestion in Humans • *Gebhard Flatz*

Perspectives in the Teaching of Human Genetics • *Ronald G. Davidson and Barton Childs*

Investigation of Genetic Linkage in Human Families • *Ray White and Jean-Marc Lalouel*

Chronic Granulomatous Disease • *John T. Curnutte and Bernard M. Babior*

Genetics of Steroid Receptors and Their Disorders • *Leonard Pinsky and Morris Kaufman*

Preface to Volume 1

During the last few years the science of human genetics has been expanding almost explosively. Original papers dealing with different aspects of the subject are appearing at an increasingly rapid rate in a very wide range of journals, and it becomes more and more difficult for the geneticist and virtually impossible for the nongeneticist to keep track of the developments. Furthermore, new observations and discoveries relevant to an overall understanding of the subject result from investigations using very diverse techniques and methodologies and originating in a variety of different disciplines. Thus, investigations in such various fields as enzymology, immunology, protein chemistry, cytology, pediatrics, neurology, internal medicine, anthropology, and mathematical and statistical genetics, to name but a few, have each contributed results and ideas of general significance to the study of human genetics. Not surprisingly it is often difficult for workers in one branch of the subject to assess and assimilate findings made in another. This can be a serious limiting factor on the rate of progress.

Thus, there appears to be a real need for critical review which summarizes the positions reached in different areas, and it is hoped that *Advances in Human Genetics* will help to meet this requirement.

Each of the contributors has been asked to write an account of the position that has been reached in the investigations of a specific topic in one of the branches of human genetics. The reviews are intended to be critical and to deal with the topic in depth from the writer's own point of view. It is hoped that the articles will provide workers in other branches of the subject, and in related disciplines, with a detailed account of the results so far obtained in the particular area, and help them to assess the relevance of these discoveries to aspects of their own work, as well as to the science as a whole. The reviews are also intended to give the reader some idea of the nature of the technical and methodological problems involved, and to indicate new directions stemming from recent advances.

The contributors have not been restricted in the arrangement or organization of their material or in the manner of its presentation, so that the reader should be able to appreciate something in the individuality of approach which goes to make up the subject of human genetics, and which, indeed, gives it much of its fascination.

HARRY HARRIS
The Galton Laboratory
University College London

KURT HIRSCHHORN
Division of Medical Genetics
Department of Pediatrics
Mount Sinai School of Medicine

Preface to Volume 10

This is the tenth volume of *Advances in Human Genetics* and some fifty different reviews covering a very wide range of topics have now appeared. Many of the earlier articles still stand as valuable sources of reference. But the subject continues to move forward at an increasing speed and its vitality is indicated by its remarkable recruitment of young investigators. New areas of research which could hardly have been envisaged only a few years ago have emerged, and quite unexpectedly discoveries have been made in parts of the subject which only recently had come to be thought as fully explored. So there continues to be a need for authoritative and critical reviews intended to keep workers in the various branches of this seemingly ever-expanding subject fully informed about the progress that is being made and also, of course, to provide a ready and accessible account of new developments in human genetics for those whose primary interests are in other fields of biological and medical research.

We see no reason to alter the general policy which was outlined in the preface to the first volume. We believe that it has served our readers well. The subject seems to us to be just as exciting and intellectually stimulating and rewarding as it did when this series was first started. We expect the next decade of research in human genetics to be as innovative and productive as the last and our aim is to record its progress in *Advances in Human Genetics*.

HARRY HARRIS
University of Pennsylvania, Philadelphia

KURT HIRSCHHORN
Mount Sinai School of Medicine
of the City University of New York

NOTE ABOUT ADDENDUM

To make the volume as up-to-date as possible, each author was given the opportunity to write a short Addendum at the time he or she received the page proofs of that particular chapter. This allows for any important new material to be presented at the latest possible time in the publication process. The Addendum is presented at the end of the book, beginning on page 201.

Contents

Chapter 1

Chorionic Villus Sampling

James D. Goldberg and Mitchell S. Golbus

Introduction 1
Early Trophoblast Development 2
Historical Perspectives 3
Techniques of Chorionic Villus Sampling 4
 Overview 4
 Transcervical Catheter Aspiration 4
 Transcervical Endoscopy 6
 Transcervical Biopsy Forceps 6
 Transabdominal Sampling 7
 Sample Processing 8
Chromosomal Analysis 8
 Direct Karyotype Analysis 8
 Karyotype Analysis of Cultured Villi 9
 Results of Karyotype Analysis 9
Metabolic Analysis of Chorionic Villi 10
 Overview 10
 Metabolic Disorders Diagnosed 12
 Pitfalls of Metabolic Diagnosis 14
DNA Analysis of Chorionic Villi 15
 Overview 15
 DNA Disorders Diagnosed 16
 Pitfalls in DNA Diagnosis of Chorionic Villi 16

Contraindications to Chorionic Villus Sampling   17
Safety of Chorionic Villus Sampling   17
Future Applications   19
References   19

Chapter 2

**The Molecular Genetics of Hemophilia A and B in Man:
Factor VIII and Factor IX Deficiency**

Stylianos E. Antonarakis

Introduction   27
Hemophilia A. Factor VIII Gene   28
    Cloning and Characterization of Factor VIII Gene
        and the Deduced Protein Sequence   28
    Mutations in the Factor VIII Gene in Hemophilia A . . .   32
    DNA Polymorphisms in the Factor VIII Gene   40
Hemophilia B. Factor IX Gene   44
    Cloning and Characterization of Factor IX Gene   44
    Mutations in the Factor IX Gene in Hemophilia B   46
    DNA Polymorphisms in the Factor IX Gene   51
X-Chromosome Mapping of Factor VIII and IX Genes . . .   53
Lessons from the Study of the Molecular Genetics of
    Hemophilia   53
References   55

Chapter 3

Cloning of the Duchenne/Becker Muscular Dystrophy Locus

Anthony P. Monaco and Louis M. Kunkel

Introduction   61
    Background Information: Clinical Aspects of DMD   62

Background Information: Biochemical Aspects
of DMD 63
Chromosomal Map Position 65
Strategies to Approach the Gene 67
Detection of Deletions in DMD and BMD Patients 71
Identification of the DMD Transcript 79
The DMD Locus 81
The DMD/BMD Protein 87
Future Prospects 91
References 92

Chapter 4

Trisomy 21: Molecular and Cytogenetic Studies of Nondisjunction

Gordon D. Stewart, Terry J. Hassold, and David M. Kurnit

Scope of the Problem 99
Problems to Be Addressed 100
    Correct and Complete Ascertainment of Parental Origin
        of Nondisjunction 100
    The Maternal Age Conundrum: Is the Maternal Age Effect
        due to Increased Production of Abnormal Eggs or
        Decreased Destruction of Abnormal Embryos? 102
    Identification of Couples at High Risk for Trisomy 21
        Offspring 104
    Is There a Correlation between Crossing Over and
        Nondisjunction on Chromosome 21? 106
    The Effect of the Parental Origin of Trisomy on the
        Phenotype of the Conceptus 109
Molecular Cytogenetic Organization of Chromosome 21:
    Implications for Studies of Nondisjunction 110
    Organization of DNA Sequences on the Short Arms
        of the Acrocentric Chromosomes 110
    The Interspersed 724 Family on the Acrocentric
        Short Arms 112

Isolation of a Large Number of Polymorphic
    Single-Copy DNA Probes That Span the Long Arm
    of Chromosome 21 118
Lessons from a Pilot Study 123
An Experimental Design to Answer the Basic Questions
    Related to Nondisjunction 126
Complete Ascertainment of Parental Origin and
    Meiotic Stage of Nondisjunction 127
The Maternal Age Conundrum: Is the Maternal Age Effect
    due to Increased Production of Abnormal Eggs or
    Decreased Destruction of Abnormal Embryos? 128
Identification of Couples at High Risk for Trisomy 21
    Offspring 129
Is There a Correlation between Crossing Over and
    Nondisjunction on Chromosome 21? 130
The Effect of the Parental Origin of Trisomy on the
    Phenotype of the Conceptus 131
Overview 132
References 133

Chapter 5

**Molecular Genetics of Human Salivary Proteins
and Their Polymorphisms**

Edwin A. Azen and Nobuyo Maeda

Introduction 141
Salivary Protein Polymorphisms 142
    Salivary Amylase (Amy) 154
    B_{12}-Binding Protein (Rs) 155
    Salivary Acid Phosphatase (s-AcP) 156
    Genetic Polymorphisms of Proline-Rich Proteins
        (PRPs) 156
    Salivary Peroxidase (SAPX) 169
    Parotid Basic Proteins (Pb) 170
    Other Polymorphisms in Human Saliva 172

Molecular Genetic Studies 172
The Proline-Rich Protein (PRP) Gene Family 172
Statherin 185
Amylase Gene Family 187
Cystatin Gene Family 189
References 191

Addendum 201

Index 205

Chapter 1

Chorionic Villus Sampling

James D. Goldberg and Mitchell S. Golbus

Reproductive Genetics Unit
Department of Obstetrics and Gynecology
University of California, San Francisco
San Francisco, California 94143

INTRODUCTION

The traditional approach to prenatal diagnosis of genetic defects has involved the use of amniocentesis at 16 menstrual weeks to obtain fetal cells for analysis. These cells are cultured for 2–4 weeks in order to provide an adequate number of cells for analysis, resulting in a prenatal diagnosis being made at 18–20 gestational weeks. If the diagnosis of an affected fetus is made, then the parents have as one option a second-trimester termination of pregnancy. This late termination of pregnancy involves increased medical risk to the mother as compared to a first-trimester termination and also causes significant psychological trauma. Because of this, efforts have been directed toward developing an earlier method of prenatal diagnosis.

Chorionic villus sampling (CVS) involves obtaining a small amount of the developing trophoblast as early as 9 menstrual weeks. This tissue is of fetal origin and can be used for a wide range of prenatal diagnostic studies. With this approach a prenatal diagnosis can be achieved in the first trimester of pregnancy. If an affected fetus is diagnosed, the couple can opt for an outpatient suction termination of pregnancy. This earlier prenatal diagnosis makes it possible to be reassured of an unaffected fetus before others need to be informed of the pregnancy. This review will discuss the development of the chorionic villus sampling procedure, its current uses, and potential applications of this new technique.

EARLY TROPHOBLAST DEVELOPMENT

In the human, fertilization of the ovum occurs most commonly in the fimbrial end of the fallopian tube or in the peritoneal cavity. By 3 days the developing embryo consists of 60 cells, 10% of which are destined to develop into the embryo and 90% of which will develop into trophoblast (Wynn, 1975). At 5 days postfertilization the blastocyst enters the uterine cavity, and is completely buried within the endometrium by day 12 (Hertig and Rock, 1941).

In preparation to receive the developing embryo the endometrium undergoes decidualization secondary to the action of increasing levels of progesterone. This decidualized endometrium is characterized by the decidua basalis in the area of trophoblast invasion, the decidua capsularis surrounding the embryo, and the decidua parietalis, which lines the rest of the uterine cavity. By 4 months gestation the decidua capsularis and parietalis fuse to obliterate the remaining uterine cavity.

Following implantation, the trophoblast differentiates into the cytotrophoblast and syncytiotrophoblast, with the syncytiotrophoblast initially invading into the decidualized endometrium and myometrium. Soon after implantation lacunae are noted in the syncytium, which coalesce and eventually become sinuses for maternal blood. Secondary villi are noted at approximately 2 weeks and are characterized by the development of a mesenchymal core. These secondary villi penetrate into maternal vessels to allow maternal blood to fill the developing lacunae. By the third week the intravillus vascular network connects with the umbilical vessels, forming a tertiary villus structure. All of the basic structures of the mature chorionic villi are essentially formed by the end of the fifth week. At this stage of gestation the chorionic villi are divided into the chorion frondosum, which is in the area of trophoblast invasion, and the chorion laeve, which surrounds the rest of the chorionic membrane. The villi in the chorion laeve will undergo degeneration as the pregnancy progresses.

HISTORICAL PERSPECTIVES

The first attempt to obtain chorionic villus was reported by Hahnemann and Mohr (1968). By using transcervical hysteroscopy, these investigators were able to obtain trophoblast from women undergoing midtrimester termination of pregnancy. Similar success in obtaining chorionic villi was reported by Kullander and Sandahl (1973). Both groups, however, reported an extremely low yield of villus material and had difficulty in culturing what little tissue they obtained. In an expanded study, Hahnemann (1974) described his attempts in 95 cases of sampling done at the time of first-trimester pregnancy termination. In 20 of these procedures visualization was extremely poor, resulting in villus samples in only four of those cases.

The first series of chorionic villus sampling (CVS) in ongoing pregnancies was a Chinese study reported in 1975 (Department of Obstetrics and Gynecology, Tietung Hospital, Anshan Iron and Steel Company, 1975). One hundred patients underwent transcervical CVS without ultrasound guidance for the prenatal diagnosis of fetal sex. Ninety-four patients were diagnosed accurately. There were four spontaneous losses reported; however, the induced termination rate was very high. This was the first study demonstrating the practical application of CVS for prenatal diagnosis. Direct tissue preparations were used for sex chromatin analysis, and thus did not contribute to solving the problem of culturing the villus material.

Also in 1975, Rhine et al. (1975) reported the ability to obtain fetal cells above the cervical mucous plug. Subsequently, (Rhine, 1977) they described the use of a specially modified, 3.5-mm plastic tube inserted above the mucous plug. With this device they obtained fetal chromosome metaphase spreads in 26% of samples. In an expanded study, Rhine and Milunsky (1979) sampled 53 patients. In

70% of the specimens fetal trophoblast was identified, but in only 49% were fetal chromosome metaphase spreads obtained. This technique was complicated by the small quantities of tissue obtained and the poor quality of the chromosome preparations.

A major advance in the analysis of chorionic villus material was reported by Niazi *et al.* (1981). These investigators devised a technique to culture chorionic villi by trypsinization and filtering to expose the inner mesenchymal core. A further advance was the report of the first direct DNA analysis of chorionic villi for prenatal diagnosis by Williamson *et al.* (1981).

These studies laid the groundwork for the use of CVS by a number of investigators in large clinical studies of ongoing pregnancies. This chapter will put into perspective the current state of chorionic villus sampling.

TECHNIQUES OF CHORIONIC VILLUS SAMPLING

Overview

A number of techniques have been used to obtain chorionic villus tissue. Most of these have involved the transcervical approach to the trophoblast. The most commonly used instrument to obtain villi has been a plastic catheter with a malleable stainless steel obturator. Other transcervical techniques used include ultrasound-directed rigid biopsy forceps and endoscopically guided biopsy forceps. A recent alternative approach to CVS has been by transabdominal aspiration. Each of these techniques, including advantages and disadvantages, warrants discussion.

Transcervical Catheter Aspiration

At present, approximately 80% of CVS procedures are performed by the transcervical catheter aspiration technique (Jackson, 1986). This involves placing the patient with a partially full bladder in the dorsal lithotomy position. The position of the trophoblast and the axis of the uterus is assessed by real-time ultrasound visualization and fetal viability is confirmed. A speculum is then inserted and the vagina is cleansed with an antiseptic solution. A tenaculum is used by many investigators to stabilize the cervix, but is not necessary in most cases. An approximately 16 gauge catheter with a malleable obturator is bent to conform to the sampling path and then inserted transcervically into the area of the chorionic villi. After removal of the internal obturator a 20 cm^3 syringe is attached and 5–10 cm^3 of negative pressure applied while withdrawing the catheter. Some investigators place a small amount of culture medium into the catheter and syringe to avoid any tissue adherence to the sidewalls. We have not found this necessary. The tissue obtained is flushed into tissue culture medium and immediately examined under a low-power dissecting microscope to verify that an adequate amount of trophoblast was obtained. As many as three passes of the catheter are performed, if necessary, with a new catheter used each time. No anesthesia is necessary. However, a cramping sensation is frequently reported by the patient as the catheter passes through the internal os of the cervix.

The initial attempts at transcervical CVS were performed without ultrasound guidance. The first objective assessment of this "blind" approach was reported by Horwell et al. (1983). Chorionic villi were obtained in 40% of 212 cases sampled prior to first-trimester termination of pregnancy. Three cases of immediate amnion rupture were noted. A follow-up study by Horwell (1984) using a longer catheter reported a somewhat higher success rate, obtaining villi in 49% of patients. A study of blind sampling by Liu et al. (1983) reported a 33% success rate of obtaining villi in 137 patients.

The use of ultrasound to guide the sampling catheter resulted in a markedly increased success rate in obtaining villi. Ward et al. (1983) reported up to a 90% success rate in obtaining trophoblast using ultrasound guidance. Rodeck et al. (1983) described a single-operator technique, with one hand holding the ultrasound transducer and the other controlling the sampling catheter. Other investigators have described similar high success rates in obtaining chorionic villi with ultrasound guidance (Old et al., 1982; Grebner et al., 1983;

Pergament *et al.*, 1983; Simoni *et al.*, 1983) and this has become the most commonly used CVS technique.

In addition to providing guidance of the catheter into the trophoblast, ultrasound provides many other advantages for CVS. One of the most important is in verifying that a fetus is viable before sampling is performed. Recent studies have shown that over 10% of women presenting for CVS have nonviable gestations (Jones *et al.*, 1986). Multiple gestations also can be identified in most instances. It must be recognized, however, that a proportion of multiple gestations observed in the first trimester will revert to a singleton gestation as pregnancy progresses (Landy *et al.*, 1986). Ultrasound also identifies local uterine variations such as fibroids or uterine contractions that can interfere with insertion and placement of the sampling catheter. Varying the fullness of the bladder is a helpful method to control the uterine axis and aid in sampling.

Transcervical Endoscopy

The use of a transcervically introduced endoscope to obtain chorionic villi has been reported by several investigators (Kazy *et al.*, 1982; Gosden *et al.*, 1982; Gustavii, 1983, 1984). This technique involves insertion of a 2.4- to 3-mm-diameter cannula through the internal os of the cervix into the uterine cavity. To enhance visualization, the uterine cavity may be distended with CO_2 or saline. After visualization of the trophoblast a sample is taken under direct vision either by a small biopsy forceps or by aspiration. Gustavii (1987) recently reported on the outcome of 100 completed pregnancies that had undergone endoscopically directed CVS. He reported a 100% success rate in obtaining tissue, with an 8% loss rate of pregnancies intended to continue.

Transcervical Biopsy Forceps

Dumez *et al.* (1985) reported on the use of an ultrasonically directed transcervical biopsy forceps. The instrument used is a rigid forceps 2 mm in diameter and 20 cm long. These investigators reported a 100% success rate in obtaining tissue. Very few other centers have tried this technique. For the centers using this approach the overall loss rate of pregnancies intended to continue has been 5.1% (Jackson, 1986).

Transabdominal Sampling

Two early reports demonstrated the feasibility of obtaining chorionic villi by the transabdominal route. Alvarez (1966) described 50 cases where a molar pregnancy was diagnosed at 10–14 menstrual weeks by transabdominal trophoblast sampling. No complications were reported in these cases. Aladjem (1969) reported obtaining 215 villus samples by transabdominal sampling in the third trimester to study placental morphology. Again, no maternal or fetal complications were reported.

The first use of transabdominal CVS for prenatal diagnosis of genetic defects was reported by Smidt-Jensen and Hahnemann (1984). Their technique used an 18-gauge, 15-cm guide needle inserted under ultrasound guidance transabdominally through the myometrium to the edge of the trophoblast. A 22 gauge, 20-cm sampling needle was then inserted into the trophoblast and a sample of chorionic villi aspirated. While tissue was obtained from every case sampled, 2–6 aspirations per patient were necessary to obtain an adequate sample. Local anesthesia was used to anesthetize the skin, but no material sedation was necessary.

Smidt-Jensen and Hahnemann (1987) recently reported their experience with 170 cases of transabdominal CVS. At the time of the report 48 of the patients were less than 28 weeks gestation and 73 had delivered. Eight patients had undergone elective termination of pregnancy and four patients had spontaneous losses. In a much smaller series, Lilford et al. (1987) reported 100% success in transabdominally obtaining tissue in 14 diagnostic cases.

While the experience with transabdominal CVS is still somewhat limited, it offers some potential benefits over the transcervical approaches. As will be discussed in the safety section of this chapter,

there have been a small number of significant maternal infections
associated with transcervical sampling. It is hoped that the transabdominal approach will lessen this risk. In addition, the implantation site in some women is very difficult to reach transcervically
due to extreme flexion of the uterus or a fundal implantation. In
these cases, the transabdominal procedure may provide much easier
access to the optimal sampling site. Potential disadvantages include
patients' fear of needles, increased discomfort, and an unknown
magnitude of risk of pregnancy loss.

Sample Processing

Immediately after sampling by any method the tissue obtained
is examined under a low-power dissecting microscope to determine
its morphology and quantity. Any maternal decidua in the sample
must be carefully dissected away. Elles has shown by analysis of
fetal and maternal DNA restriction fragment length polymorphisms
that careful identification and separation of fetal tissue in this way
results in no maternal contamination (Elles *et al.*, 1983). In most
laboratories 5–10 mg of tissue is sufficient for analysis, although for
some metabolic assays larger quantities of tissue are required. In
addition, for certain heat-sensitive metabolic assays, care must be
taken to avoid destruction of enzyme activity during sample separation.

CHROMOSOMAL ANALYSIS

Direct Karyotype Analysis

Simoni *et al.* (1983) described a method of direct chromosomal
analysis of chorionic villi based on modifications of a method reported by Evans *et al.* (1972) for the karyotyping of mouse tails.
The critical step in this method was the exposure of the tissue to
60% acetic acid to release cells from membranes. This technique
allowed the direct karyotyping of dividing cytotrophoblast cells

without the need for tissue culture. An alternative technique reported by Ford and Jahnke (1983) used collagenase to release the trophoblast cells.

One problem with the direct karyotyping procedure is the wide variation in mitotic index noted in chorionic villus tissue. Some investigators have found a marked increase in the mitotic index with short-term, 12- to 48-hr culture (Simoni, 1984; Burgoyne, 1983). Other investigators, however, have found no such increase (Ferguson-Smith and Yates, 1984). Blakemore *et al.* (1984) found that the number of mitoses was increased if the tissue was processed promptly after sampling.

A major problem with the direct method of karyotyping is the poor quality of Giemsa banding. The banding resolution is significantly decreased as compared to cultured amniocytes, which are the standard for prenatal diagnosis. Because of this, many investigators have been dissatisfied with the direct method of analysis.

Karyotype Analysis of Cultured Villi

As mentioned above, Niazi *et al.* (1981) developed a method of trypsinization and filtering to release the mesenchymal core of the chorionic villus material. An alternate method of releasing the core tissue by maceration was reported by Heaton *et al.* (1984). These released cells grow rapidly in tissue culture and have a spindle-fibroblast type of morphology. The processing and Giemsa banding of these cultured cells are similar to those for amniocytes, with a comparable level of banding resolution.

While the development of the direct method of karyotype analysis was initially thought to be a significant advance in the analysis of chorionic villus tissue, the continuing poor banding resolution has been disappointing. As new methods of improved tissue culture become available, such as enhanced culture media, *in situ* culturing, and triple-gas incubators, the analysis time of the culture method is approaching that of the direct method.

Results of Karyotype Analysis

Most CVS procedures are performed for advanced maternal age and are done in the 35- to 39-year-old maternal age group. Thus, aneuploidy rates are most accurately established for this group. Initial reports suggested a 3.4% aneuploidy rate for these patients undergoing CVS (Mikkelsen, 1985). This is double the aneuploidy rate reported at the time of amniocentesis (Golbus *et al.*, 1979) and was thought to be due to the spontaneous loss of aneuploid fetuses between the time CVS is performed and amniocentesis is done. As more patients have been sampled, the aneuploidy rate has fallen to 1.7%, which is the same as the aneuploidy rate at the time of amniocentesis (Mikkelsen, 1986). With increasing numbers of CVS procedures being performed, accurate incidence rates will become available for other chromosomal prenatal diagnostic indications.

An unexpected finding in the karyotype analysis of CVS specimens is a discrepancy between the villus karyotype and that of the fetus. In one series, this was found in 1.7% of cases and most commonly consisted of mosaicism in the villus sample for a chromosomal abnormality that was not found in subsequent fetal samples (Hogge *et al.*, 1986). In addition, there have been several reports of false-negative findings on direct chromosome preparations with subsequent aneuploidy discovered on long-term villus culture or fetal tissues (Eichenbaum *et al.*, 1986; Martin *et al.*, 1986; Linton and Lilford, 1986). Because of these findings, we currently recommend that long-term culture be performed on all villus specimens and that amniocentesis be done for confirmation in all cases of villus mosaicism.

METABOLIC ANALYSIS OF CHORIONIC VILLI

Overview

The ability to obtain and analyze chorionic villi in the first trimester of pregnancy represents a major advance in the prenatal diagnosis of inherited metabolic disease. For many of these recessive conditions the fetus carries a 25% risk of being affected, which produces considerable stress in the at-risk parents. The ability to achieve a diagnosis in the first trimester, before friends or relatives are even aware of the pregnancy, has provided many couples who had previously decided not to conceive with new reproductive options.

Several principles are especially important in the metabolic analysis of chorionic villi. Prior to attempting the prenatal diagnosis of any inherited metabolic disease, it is essential to establish or confirm the specific disorder under consideration. Efforts must be directed toward eliminating the possibility of misdiagnosis due to phenotypic, metabolic, or genetic heterogeneity. The precise enzymatic defect must be demonstrated in the proband or other affected relatives. If the proband is deceased, the heterozygosity of both parents (or of the mother, for an X-linked disease) must be documented. In all analyses for homozygosity or heterozygosity, care must be taken to demonstrate the metabolic defect using appropriate methods and reference standards from confirmed affected cases and normal controls.

The presence of the indicated enzyme must be demonstrated in normal uncultured and/or cultured chorionic villi. In addition, the possibility of tissue-specific or fetal isozymes with slightly different properties should be investigated. For each enzyme assay, optimal conditions must be established, using chorionic villi as the enzyme source. Adequate enzymatic activity must be detectable in a practical quantity of uncultured or cultured chorionic villi for the unambiguous distinction of homozygous affected and heterozygous levels.

If a specific diagnosis is undertaken for the first time by CVS, at-risk parents should be offered the options of (1) sending the specimen to a second experienced laboratory for diagnostic confirmation (perhaps by a different method) and (2) obtaining amniotic fluid cells at 16 menstrual weeks for confirmatory studies. The amniotic fluid cell studies may be particularly important if the laboratory studies of chorionic villi are inconclusive.

Following the termination of a fetus diagnosed as affected, studies should be performed to confirm the diagnosis. The use of the first-trimester suction curettage procedure not only affords the woman a safe and rapid termination without the induction of labor, but it also permits confirmation of the prenatal diagnosis by metabolic, molecular, and ultrastructural studies. In fetuses carried to

TABLE I. Disorders of Sphingolipid Metabolism

Disorder	Prenatal diagnosis[a]	Reference
Fabry	Made	Goldberg *et al.* (1985)
Farber	Feasible	Jackson (1985)
Gaucher	Made	Goldberg *et al.* (1985)
G_{M2}-Gangliosidosis	Made	Goldberg *et al.* (1985)
G_{M2}-Gangliosidosis		
Tay–Sachs: infantile	Made	Grabowski *et al.* (1984), Grebner *et al.* (1983), Pergament *et al.* (1983)
Tay–Sachs: late onset	Made	Besancon *et al.* (1984)
Sandhoff disease	Feasible	Jackson (1985)
Krabbe	Made	Kleijer *et al.* (1984a)
Mucolipidosis IV	Feasible	Simoni *et al.* (1983)
Metachromatic leukodystrophy	Made	Goldberg *et al.* (1985)
Multiple sulfatase deficiency	Made	Jackson (1985)
Niemann–Pick	Made	Goldberg *et al.* (1985)

[a] Made: Indicates that the prenatal diagnosis has been accomplished and confirmed. Feasible: Indicates that the specific enzyme activity has been demonstrated in chorionic villi, but no affected diagnosis has been made.

term the diagnosis also should be confirmed by obtaining placental tissue, amnion, and/or cord blood at delivery.

Metabolic Disorders Diagnosed

The metabolic disorders that have been diagnosed by CVS are listed in Tables I–VII. Disorders for which the deficient enzyme has

TABLE II. Disorders of Neutral Lipid Metabolism

Disorder	Prenatal diagnosis[a]	Reference
Adrenoleukodystrophy	Made	Boué *et al.* (1985)
Wolman	Feasible	Jackson (1985)
Zellweger syndrome	Made	Hajra *et al.* (1985), Schutgens *et al.* (1984)

[a] See footnote to Table I.

TABLE III. Disorders of Glycoprotein Metabolism

Disorder	Prenatal diagnosis[a]	Reference
Fucosidosis	Feasible	Poenaru et al. (1984a, 1985), Beyer and Wiederschain (1984)
Mannosidosis	Feasible	Poenaru et al. (1984b, 1985)
Mucolipidosis II	Made	Poenaru et al. (1984a)
Galactosialidosis	Feasible	Simoni et al. (1983)

[a] See footnote to Table I.

TABLE IV. Disorders of Mucopolysaccharide Metabolism

Disorder[a]	Prenatal diagnosis[b]	Reference
MPS I (Hurler)	Made	Jackson (1985), Simoni et al. (1984)
MPS II (Hunter)	Made	Kleijer et al. (1984b), Harper et al. (1984), Lykkelund et al. (1983)
MPS IIIA (Sanfillipo A)	Made	Kleijer et al. (1986)
MPS IIIB (Sanfillipo B)	Feasible	Marsh and Fensom (1985)
MPS VII	Feasible	Kazy et al. (1982), Simoni et al. (1983), Poenoru et al. (1984b)

[a] MPS, Mucopolysaccharidosis.
[b] See footnote to Table I.

TABLE V. Disorders of the Urea Cycle Constituents

Disorder	Prenatal diagnosis[a]	Reference
Argininosuccinic acidemia	Feasible	Vimal et al. (1984)
Citrullinemia	Made	Kleijer et al. (1984c)

[a] See footnote to Table I.

TABLE VI. Disorders of Propionate and Methylmalonate Metabolism

Disorder	Prenatal diagnosis[a]	Reference
Propionic acidemia	Feasible	Sweetman et al. (1986)
3-Methylcrotonylglycinuria	Feasible	Sweetman et al. (1986)
Methylmalonic acidemia	Feasible	Kleijer et al. (1984c)
Pyruvate carboxylase deficiency	Feasible	Sweetman et al. (1986)
Multiple carboxylase deficiency	Feasible	Sweetman et al. (1986)
4-Hydroxybutyric aciduria	Feasible	Sweetman et al. (1986)
4-Amino-butyric acid aminotransferase deficiency	Feasible	Sweetman et al. (1986)

[a] See footnote to Table I.

been demonstrated to be present in chorionic villi and are thus feasible for prenatal diagnosis are also listed.

Pitfalls of Metabolic Diagnosis

The major pitfall in the analysis of uncultured or cultured chorionic villi is maternal contamination. This occurs during the sam-

TABLE VII. Other Disorders

Disorder	Prenatal diagnosis[a]	Reference
Glycogen storage disease type II	Made	Jackson (1985)
Maple-syrup urine disease	Feasible	Jackson (1985)
Homocystinuria	Made	Goldberg et al. (1985)
Cystinosis	Made	Jackson (1985)
Tyrosinemia	Feasible	Holme et al. (1985), Kvittingen et al. (1986)
Lesch–Nyhan	Made	Gibbs et al. (1984)
Severe combined immune deficiency (adenosine deaminase deficient)	Feasible	Simoni et al. (1983)
Menkes	Made	Tonneson et al. (1985)
X-linked ichthyosis	Feasible	Lan et al. (1984)
Glucose phosphate isomerase deficiency	Feasible	Dallapiccola et al. (1986)
Galactosemia	Made	Kleijer et al. (1986)
Hypophosphatasia	Made	Warren et al. (1985)

[a] See footnote to Table I.

TABLE VIII. First-Trimester Metabolic Prenatal Diagnosis Discrepancies

Disease[a]	Direct CV	Cultured cells[b]	Fetus
MPS I	Not affected	AF: Affected	Affected
MPS I	Affected	AF: Not affected	Not affected
MPS I	Affected	AF: Not affected	Not affected
MPS I	Affected	AF: Not affected	Not affected
MLD	Affected	CV: Affected; AF: not affected	Not affected
MLD	Inconclusive	—	Normal[c]
MPS IIIA	Affected	CV: Not affected	Affected

[a] MPS, Mucopolysaccharidosis. MLD, Metachromatic leukodystrophy.
[b] AF, amniotic fluid. CV, chorionic villi.
[c] Couple elected to terminate, rather than await subsequent studies.

pling procedure, when fragments of maternal decidua may be aspirated with the villus material. Great care must be taken in sample preparation to carefully dissect away any contaminating decidua, using a low-power dissecting microscope. Attention must be paid to the heat generated by the microscope light source to avoid inactivating heat-labile enzymes.

Discrepancies have occurred in the diagnostic evaluation of several fetuses, as listed in Table VIII (Goldberg *et al.*, 1985). These discrepancies may have resulted from a variety of causes, including (1) failure to optimize assay conditions for chorionic villus analysis, (2) maternal contamination, and (3) investigator inexperience with a particular assay.

DNA ANALYSIS OF CHORIONIC VILLI

Overview

Chorionic villi have proven to be an excellent tissue source for the extraction of DNA for the molecular diagnosis of genetic disease. The list of disorders diagnosable by DNA analysis is rapidly growing and all are feasible by chorionic villus analysis. It is possible to obtain an average of 30 μg of DNA per direct chorionic villus sample,

TABLE IX. DNA Analysis of Chorionic Villi

Disorder	Prenatal diagnosis[a]	Reference
Myotonic dystrophy	Feasible	Lunt et al. (1986)
Autosomal dominant polycystic kidney disease	Made	Reeders et al. (1986)
Fetal-sex determination	Made	Gosden et al. (1984)
Cystic fibrosis	Made	Farrall et al. (1986)
β-Thalassemia	Made	Rosatelle et al. (1985), Old et al. (1982)
Adrenoleukodystrophy	Made	Boué et al. (1985)
Hemophilia A	Feasible	Gitschier et al. (1985), Tonnesen et al. (1984b)
Sickle cell	Made	Goossens et al. (1983)
Hemophilia B	Feasible	Tonnesen et al. (1984a)
α-Thalassemia	Made	Wang et al. (1986)

[a] See footnote to Table I.

which provides adequate material for five or six restriction enzyme digestions.

DNA Disorders Diagnosed

The disorders that have been attempted or diagnosed by CVS in the first trimester are listed in Table IX. As mentioned above, this list is rapidly expanding.

Pitfalls in DNA Diagnosis of Chorionic Villi

Prenatal diagnoses using chorionic villi and recombinant DNA technology have the same pitfalls as any type of prenatal molecular analysis. These include: (1) maternal contamination of the DNA, (2) probe contamination, (3) technical difficulties, such as incomplete restriction digestion, (4) meiotic crossover when linkage analysis is being used, and (5) nonpaternity.

CONTRAINDICATIONS TO CHORIONIC VILLUS SAMPLING

There are several relative contraindications to chorionic villus sampling. The first is advanced gestational age. An increased loss rate has been demonstrated when transcervical CVS is performed beyond 12 weeks gestation (Hogge *et al.,* 1986). Active vaginal bleeding is also a contraindication to CVS, in that it may indicate an impending miscarriage. Some centers performing CVS have considered multiple gestations to be a contraindication to the procedure. These centers are concerned that only one fetus might be sampled, resulting in a misdiagnosis in the nonsampled fetus. As more multiple gestations are sampled, the accuracy and risk of this approach will become clearer.

Several contraindications apply only to the transcervical techniques of CVS. These include: (1) active cervical infection, herpes, or gonorrhea, (2) uterine fibroids preventing passage of the sampling catheter, and (3) cervical stenosis.

SAFETY OF CHORIONIC VILLUS SAMPLING

The primary concern with any new technique is its safety. This has been particularly difficult to assess with CVS because of the significant baseline fetal loss rate at this gestational age. Until recently the fetal loss rate following the demonstration of fetal heart activity at 8–9 menstrual weeks was unknown. Two recent studies are summarized in Table X (Wilson *et al.,* 1984; Gilmore and

TABLE X. Risk of Spontaneous Abortion

Investigators	Number	Risk at given maternal age, %			
		<30	30–34	35–39	≥40 years
Wilson *et al.* (1984)	734	1.5	2.5	4.5	—
Gilmore and McNay (1985)	1960	1.7	2.5	2.6	13.6

McNay, 1985). Both of these studies reveal an increasing fetal loss rate with increasing maternal age. In the maternal age range where CVS is most commonly performed ($\geq$35 years) baseline fetal loss rate was 4.1–4.5%.

These baseline loss figures must be compared to the fetal loss rate following CVS. The most comprehensive collection of fetal loss data has been collected in the *CVS Latest Newsletter* (Jackson, 1986). This newsletter reports results from contributors worldwide and currently lists over 20,000 procedures. The overall loss rate has remained stable at approximately 4%. Comparison of this to the baseline loss rate of 4.1–4.5%, indicates a very small procedure-related loss rate. Increased numbers of cases will be needed to assess this risk more accurately.

To assess this loss rate in a more controlled manner, several countries have undertaken studies to compare the safety and accuracy of CVS as compared to amniocentesis, including a seven-center collaborative study sponsored by the National Institute of Child Health and Human Development. This study has been designed as a case–control study to assess both the accuracy and safety of CVS as compared to amniocentesis. Other studies underway in Canada and several Scandinavian and European centers are being conducted in a randomized manner and will provide valuable safety information.

Beside fetal loss, other areas of safety are of importance. There have been several maternal infections associated with the transcervical CVS procedure. In a recent review of 1000 consecutive cases of CVS at the University of California at San Francisco the maternal infection rate was 0.6% (Hogge *et al.,* 1986). One case resulted in an extremely severe infection, leading to septic shock and the need for hysterectomy (Barela *et al.,* 1986).

Rupture of the membranes following the procedure has been reported in a small number of cases, as has oligohydramnios without rupture of the membranes. Results from the many collaborative studies will be needed to assess the magnitude of risk of these complications.

FUTURE APPLICATIONS

The emergence of CVS as a method for prenatal diagnosis in the first trimester of pregnancy should have benefits for fetal treatment efforts by making possible earlier intervention or possibly even prevention of certain fetal diseases. To date, there has been limited experience with these approaches, but initial reports have been encouraging.

Two recently reported cases demonstrate the possibility of successful *in utero* therapy of disorders resulting from alteration in fetal hormone concentration. To prevent masculinization of fetuses at risk for congenital adrenal hyperplasia, David and Forest (1984) attempted to suppress the fetal adrenal gland by maternal administration of steroids. In the first case, oral administration of maternal hydrocortisone was begun at 6.5 menstrual weeks. Fetal adrenal suppression, however, was not complete and a partially masculinized female fetus was born. In a second case, administration of dexamethasone to the mother was begun at 5 menstrual weeks, with amniocentesis at 15 weeks confirming adrenal suppression and predicting an affected female fetus. Neonatal evaluation confirmed 21-hydroxylase deficiency with no evidence of masculinization. CVS would potentially allow the diagnosis of an affected female fetus to be made before masculinization begins in the first trimester, and thus avoid the unnecessary treatment of an unaffected or male fetus.

As more disorders become amenable to *in utero* therapy CVS will provide important early diagnostic information. If a fetus is diagnosed to be normal at this stage of pregnancy, therapy can be avoided, eliminating any potential harmful side effects of prolonged administration of the therapeutic agent.

REFERENCES

Aladjem, S., 1969, Fetal assessment through biopsy of the human placenta, in: *The Fetoplacental Unit* (A. Pecile and C. Finzi, eds.), pp. 392–402, Excerpta Medica Foundation, Amsterdam.

Alvarez, H., 1966, Diagnosis of hydatidiform mole by transabdominal placental biopsy, *Am. J. Obstet. Gynecol.* **95**:538–541.

Barela, A. I., Kleinman, G. E., Golditch, I. M., Menke, D. J., Hogge, W. A., and Golbus, M. S., 1986, Septic shock with renal failure after chorionic villus sampling, *Am. J. Obstet. Gynecol.* **154**:1100–1102.

Besancon, A. M., Belon, J. P., Castelnau, L., Dumez, Y., and Poenaru, L., 1984, Prenatal diagnosis of atypical Tay–Sachs disease by chorionic villi sampling, *Prenat. Diagn.* **4**:365–370.

Beyer, E. M., and Wiederschain, G., 1984, Activity and multiple forms of alpha-L-fucosidase and hexodaminidase in chorion biopsy specimens and some fetal organs, *Prenat. Diagn.* **4**:43–49.

Blakemore, K. J., Watson, M. S., Samuelson, J., Breg, W. R., and Mahoney, M. J., 1984, A method of processing first-trimester chorionic villous biopsies for cytogenetic analysis, *Am. J. Hum Genet.* **36**:1386–1393.

Boué, J., Oberlé, I., Heilig, R., Mandel, J. L., Moser, A., Moser, H., Larsen, J. W., Dumez, Y., and Boué, A., 1985, First trimester prenatal diagnosis of adrenoleukodystrophy by determination of very long chain fatty acid levels and by linkage analysis to a DNA probe, *Hum. Genet.* **69**:272–274.

Burgoyne, P., 1983, Direct chromosome preparations from chorionic villi, *Prenat. Diagn. Group News.* **7**:3–4.

Dallapiccola, B., Novelli, G., Ferranti, G., Pachi, A., Cristiani, M. L., and Magnani, M., 1986, First trimester monitoring of a pregnancy at risk for glucose phosphate isomerase deficiency, *Prenat. Diagn.* **6**:101–107.

David, M., and Forest, M. G., 1984, Prenatal treatment of congenital adrenal hyperplasia resulting from 21-hydroxylase deficiency, *J. Pediatr.* **105**:799–803.

Department of Obstetrics and Gynecology, Tietung Hospital, Anshan Iron and Steel Company, 1975, Fetal sex prediction by sex chromatin of chorionic villi cells during early pregnancy, *Chin. Med. J.* **1**:117–126.

Dumez, Y., Goossens, M., Boué, J., Poenaru, L., Dommergues, M., and Henrion, R., 1985, Chorionic sampling using rigid forceps under ultrasound control, in: *First Trimester Fetal Diagnosis* (M. Fraccaro *et al.*, eds.), pp. 38–45, Springer-Verlag, Berlin.

Eichenbaum, S. Z., Krumins, E. J., Fortune, D. W., and Duke, J., 1986, False-negative finding on chorionic villus sampling, *Lancet* **2**:391.

Elles, R. G., Williamson, R., Niazi, M., Coleman, D. V., and Horwell, D. H., 1983, Absence of maternal contamination of chorionic villi used for fetal-gene analysis, *N. Engl. J. Med.* **308**:1433–1435.

Evans, E. P., Burtenshaw, M. D., and Ford, C. E., 1972, Chromosomes of mouse embryos and newborn young: Preparations from membranes and tail tips, *Stain Technol.* **47**:229–234.

Farrall, M., Law, H.-Y., Rodeck, Ch. H., Warren, R., Stanier, P., Super, M., Lissens, W., Scambler, P., Watson, E., Wainwright, B., and Williamson, R., 1986, First trimester prenatal diagnosis of cystic fibrosis with linked DNA probes, *Lancet* **2**:1402–1405.

Ferguson-Smith, M. A., and Yates, J. R. W., 1984, Maternal age specific rates for chromosome aberrations and factors influencing them. Report of a collaborative study on 52,965 amniocenteses, *Prenat. Diagn.* **4**:5–44.

Ford, J. H., and Jahnke, A. B., 1983, Handling chorionic villi for direct chromosome studies, *Lancet* **2**:1491–1492.

Gibbs, D. A., McFadyen, I. R., Crawfurd, M. A., Keizer, E. E. M., Headhouse-Benson, C. N., Wilson, T. M., and Farrant, P. H., 1984, First trimester diagnosis of Lesch–Nyhan syndrome, *Lancet* **2**:1180–1183.

Gilmore, D. H., and McNay, M. B., 1985, Spontaneous fetal loss rate in early pregnancy, *Lancet* **1**:107.

Gitschier, J., Lawn, R. M., Rotblat, F., Goldman, E., and Tuddenham, E. G. D., 1985, Antenatal diagnosis and carrier detection of haemophilia A using factor VIII gene probe, *Lancet* **1**:1093–1094.

Golbus, M. S., Loughman, W. D., Epstein, C. J., Halbasch, G., Stephens, J. D., and Hall, B. D., 1979, Prenatal genetic diagnosis in 3000 amniocenteses, *N. Engl. J. Med.* **300**:157–163.

Goldberg, J. D., Grabowski, G. A., Driscoll, M. C., Gordon, R. E., Berkowitz, R. L., and Desnick, R. J., 1985, First trimester fetal diagnosis: Principles and potential pitfalls in enzymatic and molecular diagnoses, in: *First Trimester Fetal Diagnosis* (M. Fraccaro *et al.*, eds.), pp. 218–234, Springer-Verlag, Berlin.

Goossens, M., Dumez, Y., Kaplan, L., Lupker, M., Chabret, C., Henrion, R., and Rosa, J., 1983, Prenatal diagnosis of sickle-cell anemia in the first trimester of pregnancy, *N. Engl. J. Med.* **309**:831–833.

Gosden, J. R., Mitchell, A. R., Gosden, C. M., Rodeck, C. H., and Morsman, J. M., 1982, Direct vision chorion biopsy and chromosome-specific DNA probes for determination of fetal sex in first-trimester prenatal diagnosis, *Lancet* **2**:1416–1419.

Gosden, J. R., Gosden, C. M., Christie, S., Morsman, J. M., and Rodeck, C. H., 1984, Rapid fetal sex determination in first trimester prenatal diagnosis by dot hybridisation of DNA probes, *Lancet* **1**:540–541.

Grabowski, G. A., Kruse, J. R., Goldberg, J. D., Chockkalingam, K., Gordon, R. E., Blakemore, K. J., Mahoney, M. J., and Desnick, R. J., 1984, First trimester prenatal diagnosis of Tay–Sachs disease, *Am. J. Hum Genet.* **36**:1369–1378.

Grebner, E. E., Wapner, R. J., Barr, M. A., and Jackson, L. G., 1983, Prenatal Tay–Sachs diagnosis by chorionic villi sampling, *Lancet* **2**:286–287.

Gustavii, B., 1983, First trimester chromosomal analysis of chorionic villi obtained by direct vision technique, *Lancet* **2**:507–508.

Gustavii, B., 1984, Chorionic biopsy and miscarriage in first trimester, *Lancet* **1**:562.

Gustavii, B., 1987, Endoscopic chorion villus sampling, in: *Chorion Villus Sampling* (E. M. Symonds and M. S. Golbus, eds.), pp. 137–141, Chapman and Hall, London.

Hahnemann, N., 1974, Early prenatal diagnosis; a study of biopsy techniques and cell culturing from extraembryonic membranes, *Clin. Genet.* **6**:294–306.

Hahnemann, N., and Mohr, J., 1968, Genetic diagnosis in the embryo by means of biopsy from extraembryonic membranes, *Bull. Eur. Soc. Hum. Genet.* **2**:23–29.

Hajra, A. K., Datta, N. S., Jackson, L. G., Moser, A. B., Moser, H. W., Larsen, J. W., and Powers, J., 1985, Prenatal diagnosis of Zellweger cerebrohepatorenal syndrome, *N. Engl. J. Med.* **312**:445–446.

Harper, P. S., Bamforth, S., Rees, D., and Upadhyaya, 1984, Chorion biopsy for prenatal testing in Hunter's syndrome, *Lancet* **2**:812–813.

Heaton, D. E., Czepulkowski, B. H., Horwell, D. H., and Coleman, D. V., 1984,

Chromosome analysis of first trimester chorionic villus biopsies prepared by a
maceration technique, *Prenat. Diagn.* 4:279–287.

Hertig, A. T., and Rock, J., 1941, Two human ova of the pre-villous stage having an
ovulation age of about eleven and twelve days respectively, *Contrib. Embryol.
Carnegie Inst.* 29:127–156.

Hogge, W. A., Schonberg, S. A., and Golbus, M. S., 1986, Chorionic villus sampling:
Experience of the first 1000 cases, *Am. J. Obstet. Gynecol.* 154:1249–1252.

Holme, E., Lindblad, B., and Lindstedt, S., 1985, Possibilities for treatment and for
early prenatal diagnosis of hereditary tyrosinaemia, *Lancet* 1:527.

Horwell, D. H., 1984, Further experience with chorionic villus aspiration, *J. Obstet.
Gynecol.* 5:66.

Horwell, D. H., Loeffler, F. E., and Coleman, D. V., 1983, Assessment of a transcervical aspiration technique for chorionic villus biopsy in the first trimester of
pregnancy, *Br. J. Obstet. Gynaecol.* 90:196–198.

Jackson, L. (ed.), 1985, *CVS Latest News* (Jefferson Medical College, Philadelphia),
1985(February 5).

Jackson, L. (ed.), 1986, *CVS Latest News* (Jefferson Medical College, Philadelphia),
1986(September 12).

Jones, S., Dorfmann, A., Patton, L., Pitt, C., Joyce, B., Sigler, M. E., Fleming, G.,
Rosen, L., and Schulman, J. D., 1986, Non-viable pregnancy in patients antic-
ipating chorionic villus sampling, *Am. J. Hum. Genet.* 34:A257.

Kazy, Z., Rozovsky, I. S., Bakharev, V. A., 1982, Chorion biopsy in early pregnancy:
A method of early prenatal diagnosis of inherited disorders, *Prenat. Diagn.* 2:39–
45.

Kleijer, W. J., Mancini, G. M. S., Jahoda, M. G. J., Vosters, R. P. L., Sachs, E.
S., Niermeijer, M. F., and Galjaard, H., 1984a, First trimester diagnosis of
Krabbe's disease by direct enzyme analysis of chorionic villi, *N. Engl. J. Med.*
311:1257.

Kleijer, W. J., Van Diggelen, O. P., Janse, H. C., Galjaard, H., Dumez, Y., and
Boué, J., 1984b, First trimester diagnosis of Hunter syndrome on chorionic villi,
Lancet 2:472.

Kleijer, W. J., Thoomes, R., Galjaard, H., Wendel, U., and Fowler, B., 1984c, First
trimester (chorion biopsy) diagnosis of citrullinaemia and methylmalonicaciduria,
Lancet 2:1340.

Kleijer, W. J., Janse, H. C., Vosters, R. P., Niermeijer, M. F., and van de Kamp,
J. J., 1986, First-trimester diagnosis of mucopolysaccharidosis IIIA (Sanfillipo
A disease), *N. Engl. J. Med.* 314:185–186.

Kullander, S., and Sandahl, B., 1973, Fetal chromosome analysis after transcervical
placental biopsies during early pregnancy, *Acta Obstet. Gynaecol. Scand.*
52:355–359.

Kvittingen, E. A., Guibaud, P. P., Divry, P., Mandon, G., Rolland, M. O., Domenich,
Y., Jakobs, C., and Christen, E., 1986, Prenatal diagnosis of hereditary tyrosinaemia type I by determination of fumarylacetoacetase in chorionic villus material, *Eur. J. Pediatr.* 144:597–598.

Lam, S. T. S., Fensom, A. H., Coleman, D., Heaton, D., Morsman, J., Nicolaides,
K., and Rodeck, C. H., 1984, Steroid sylphatase activity in trophoblast samples,
J. Obstet. Gynaecol. 5:24–26.

Landy, H. L., Weiner, S., Corson, S. L., Batzer, F. R., and Bolognese, R. J., 1986,

The "vanishing twin". Ultrasonographic assessment of disappearance in the first trimester, *Am. J. Obstet. Gynecol.* **155:**14–19.

Lilford, R. J., Linton, G., Irving, H. C., Groves, J., Mason, M. K., Crompton, A. C., and Maxwell, D., 1987, Development and clinical application, in: *Chorion Villus Sampling* (E. M. Symonds and M. S. Golbus, eds.), pp. 160–171, Chapman and Hall, London.

Linton, G., and Lilford, R. J., 1986, False-negative finding on chorionic villus sampling, *Lancet* **2:**630.

Liu, D. T. Y., Mitchell, J., Johnson, J., and Wass, D. M., 1983, Trophoblast sampling by blind transcervical aspiration, *Br. J. Obstet. Gynaecol.* **90:**1119–1123.

Lunt, P. W., Meredith, A. L., and Harper, P. S., 1986, First-trimester prediction in fetus at risk for myotonic distrophy, *Lancet* **2:**350–351.

Lykkelund, C., Sondergaard, F., Therkelsen, A. J., Tonnesen, T., Rasmussen, V., Mikkelsen, M., Guttler, F., and Nyland, M. H., 1983, Feasibility of first trimester prenatal diagnosis of Hunter syndrome, *Lancet* **2:**1147.

Marsh, J., and Fensom, A. H., 1985, 4-Methylumbelliferyl alpha-*N*-acetylglucosaminidase activity for diagnosis of Sanfillipo B disease, *Clin. Genet.* **27:**258–262.

Martin, A., Elias, S., Rosinsky, B., Bombard, A., and Simpson, J., 1986, False-negative finding on chorionic villus sampling, *Lancet* **2:**391–392.

Mikkelsen, M., 1985, Cytogenetic findings in first trimester chorionic villi biopsies: A collaborative study, in: *First Trimester Fetal Diagnosis* (M. Fraccaro *et al.*, eds.), pp. 109–120, Springer-Verlag, Berlin.

Mikkelsen, M., 1986, Presented at 7th International Congress of Human Genetics, Berlin.

Niazi, M., Coleman, D. V., and Loeffler, F. E., 1981, Trophoblast sampling in early pregnancy. Culture of rapidly dividing cells from immature placental villi, *Br. J. Obstet. Gynaecol.* **88:**1081–1085.

Old, J. M., Ward, R. H. T., Karagozlu, F., Petrou, M., and Modell, B, 1982, First trimester fetal diagnosis for haemoglobinopathies: Three cases, *Lancet* **2:**1413–1416.

Pergament, E., Ginsberg, N., Verlinsky, Y., Cadkin, A., Chu, L., and Trnka, L., 1983, Prenatal Tay–Sachs diagnosis by chorionic villi sampling, *Lancet* **2:**286–287.

Poenaru, L., Castelnau, L., Dumez, Y., and Thepot, F., 1984a, First trimester prenatal diagnosis of mucolipidosis II (I-cell disease) by choiotic biopsy, *Am. J. Hum. Genet.* **36:**1379–1385.

Poenaru, L., Kaplan, L., Dumez, Y., and Dreyfuss, J. C., 1984b, Evaluation of possible first trimester prenatal diagnosis in lysosomal diseases by trophoblast biopsy, *Pediatr. Res.* **18:**1032–1034.

Poenaru, L., Castelnau, L., Choiset, A., Rouquet, Y., and Thepot, F., 1985, Lysosomal hydrolase activity in chorionic villi and embryonic cells in culture, *Hum. Genet.* **69:**378–379.

Reeders, S. T., Zerres, K., Gal, A., Hogenkamp, T., Propping, P., Schmidt, W., Waldherr, R., Dolata, M. M., Davies, K. E., and Weatherall, D. J., 1986, Prenatal diagnosis of autosomal dominant polycystic kidney disease with a DNA probe, *Lancet* **2:**6–8.

Rhine, S. A., and Milunsky, A., 1979, Utilization of trophoblast for early prenatal diagnosis, in: *Genetic Disorders and the Fetus* (A. Milunsky, ed.), pp. 536–537, Plenum Press, New York.

Rhine, S. A., Cain, J. L., Cleary, R. E., Palmer, C. G., and Thompson, J. F., 1975, Prenatal sex detection with endocervical smears: Successful results using Y body fluorescence, *Am. J. Obstet. Gynecol.* **122**:155–160.

Rhine, S. A., Palmer, C. G., and Thompson, J. F., 1977, A simple first trimester alternative to amniocentesis for prenatal diagnosis, *Birth Defects Orig. Art. Ser.* **12**:(3D):231–247.

Rodeck, C. H., Morsman, J. M., Gosden, C. M., and Gosden, J. R., 1983, Development of an improved technique for first-trimester microsampling of chorion, *Br. J. Obstet. Gynaecol.* **90**:1113–1118.

Rosatelli, C., Falchi, A. M., Tuveri, T., Scalas, M. T., Di Tucci, A., Monni, G., and Cao, A., 1985, Prenatal diagnosis of beta-thalassemia with the synthetic-oligomer technique, *Lancet* **1**:241–243.

Schutgens, R. B. H., Heymans, H. S. A., Wanders, R. J. A., Bosch, H. V. D., and Schrakamp, G., 1984, Prenatal detection of Zellweger syndrome, *Lancet* **2**:1339–1340.

Simoni, G., 1984, The cytogenetics of first trimester fetal diagnosis, International Symposium on First Trimester Fetal Diagnosis, Rapallo.

Simoni, G., Brambati, B., Danesino, C., Rossella, F., Terzoli, G. L., Ferrari, M., and Fraccaro, M., 1983, Efficient direct chromosome analyses and enzyme determinations from chorionic villi samples in the first trimester of pregnancy, *Hum. Genet.* **63**:349–357.

Simoni, G., Brambati, B., Danesino, C., Terzoli, G. L., Romitti, L., Rosella, F., and Fraccaro, M., 1984, Diagnostic application of first trimester trophoblast sampling in 100 pregnancies, *Hum. Genet.* **66**:252–259.

Smidt-Jensen, S., and Hahnemann, N., 1984, Transabdominal fine needle biopsy from chorionic villi in the first trimester, *Prenat. Diagn.* **4**:163–169.

Smidt-Jensen, S., and Hahnemann, N., 1987, Danish experience, in: *Chorion Villus Sampling* (E. M. Symonds and M. S. Golbus, eds.), pp. 145–159, Chapman and Hall, London.

Sweetman, F. R., Gibson, K. M., Sweetman, L., Nyhan, W. L., Chin, H., Swartz, W., and Jones, O. W., 1986, Activity of biotin-dependent and GABA metabolizing enzymes in chorionic villus samples: Potential for first trimester prenatal diagnosis, *Prenat. Diagn.* **6**:187–194.

Tonnesen, T., Sondergaard, F., Güttler, F., Oberlé, I., Moisan, J. P., Mandel, J. L., Hauge, M., and Damsgaard, E. M., 1984a, Exclusion of haemophilia B in male fetus by chorionic villus biopsy, *Lancet* **2**:932.

Tonnesen, T., Sondergaard, F., Mikkelsen, M., Davies, K. E., Old, J., Winter, R. M., and Hauge, M., 1984b, X-chromosome-specific probe DX13 for carrier detection and first trimester prenatal diagnosis in haemophilia A, *Lancet* **2**:1269–1270.

Tonnesen, T., Horn, N., Sondergaard, F., Mikkelsen, M., Boué, J., Damsgaard, E., and Heydorn, K., 1985, Measurement of copper in chorionic villi for the first trimester diagnosis of Menkes' disease, *Lancet* **1**:1038–1039.

Vimal, C. M., Fensom, A. H., Heaton, D., Ward, R. H. T., Garrod, P., and Penketh, R. J. A., 1984, Prenatal diagnosis of argininosuccinicaciduria by analysis of cultured chorionic villi, *Lancet* **2**:521–522.

Wang, L. M., Zhang, J. W., Wu, G. Y., Wang, S. W., Fan, Y., Huang, Y., Zhao, L., Wang, R., Su, J., Zhang, N., Long, G., Li, Q., Zou, P., Liang, R., and Liang, Z., 1986, First-trimester prenatal diagnosis of severe alpha-thalassemia, *Prenat. Diagn.* **6:**89–95.

Ward, R. H. T., Modell, B., Petrou, M., Karagozlu, F., and Douratsos, E., 1983, Method of sampling chorionic villi in first trimester of pregnancy under guidance of real time ultrasound, *Br. Med. J.* **286:**1542.

Warren, R. C., McKenzie, C. F., Rodeck, C. H., Moscoso, G., Brock, D. J. H., and Barrow, L., 1985, First trimester diagnosis of hypophosphatasia with a monoclonal antibody to the liver/bone/kidney isoenzyme of alkaline phosphatase, *Lancet* **2:**856–858.

Williamson, R., Eskdale, J., Coleman, D. V., Niazi, M., Loeffler, F. E., and Modell, B. M., 1981, Direct gene analysis of chorionic villi: A possible technique for first trimester antenatal diagnosis of haemoglobinopathies, *Lancet* **2:**1125–1127.

Wilson, R. D., Kendrick, V., Wittmann, B. K., and McGillivray, B. C., 1984, Risk of spontaneous abortion in ultrasonically normal pregnancies, *Lancet* **2:**920–921.

Wynn, R. M., 1975, Development and ultrastructural adaptions of the human placenta, *Eur. J. Gynaecol. Reprod. Biol.* **5:**3–21.

Chapter 2

The Molecular Genetics of Hemophilia A and B in Man

Factor VIII and Factor IX Deficiency

Stylianos E. Antonarakis

Genetics Unit
Department of Pediatrics
The Johns Hopkins University School of Medicine
Baltimore, Maryland 21205

INTRODUCTION

Hemophilias are relatively common inherited disorders of blood co-agulation arising from deficiency of two different clotting factors VIII and IX. Hemophilia A, or classic hemophilia, is associated with abnormality of factor VIII and affects about 1 in every 10,000 males; hemophilia B, or Christmas disease, is associated with abnormality of factor IX and affects about 1 in every 50,000 males (McKee, 1983). Both factors are involved in the middle phase of the intrinsic clotting cascade, which consists of several inactive proteases and cofactors that are serially activated in response to an initial stimulus. The end product of the cascade is the production of the insoluble fibrin from the soluble protein fibrinogen. Fibrin then forms a filamentous net-work and stabilizes the platelet plug. Factor IX is a serine protease, which after proteolytic cleavage by factor XIa becomes activated (IXa) and with the help of factor VIII:Ca, Ca^{2+}, and phospholipid activates factor X. Factor VIII in its "activated" form VIII:Ca is actually a cofactor for the activation of factor X [see Jackson and Nemerson (1980) for review].

Hemophilias A and B exhibit similar phenotypes (clinical pictures), mainly prolonged bleeding after minor trauma. The differential diagnosis depends on laboratory clotting tests to distinguish between the two defects (Ratnoff, 1960). Both disorders are inherited as X-chromosome-linked conditions, with affected males and female carriers of the abnormal genes.

In this review the recent advances in the molecular characterization of the hemophilias will be discussed. The cloning and characterization of both factor VIII and IX genes, the description of DNA polymorphism markers associated with these genes, and recent advances in the molecular pathology of hemophilias have provided a better understanding of the pathogenesis of these disorders and facilitated the detection of carriers and the prenatal diagnosis.

HEMOPHILIA A. FACTOR VIII GENE

Cloning and Characterization of Factor VIII Gene and the Deduced Protein Sequence

In 1984 researchers in two biotechnology companies (Genentech and Genetics Institute) reported the cloning of human factor VIII gene (Gitschier *et al.*, 1984; Toole *et al.*, 1984; Wood *et al.*, 1984). Both groups used synthetic oligonucleotides as probes to clone and characterize the factor VIII gene from genomic and cDNA libraries. The oligonucleotide sequences used were deduced from small sequenced peptides of the human and porcine factor VIII (Vehar *et al.*, 1984; Fass *et al.*, 1982). The entire gene spans 186 kilobases (kb) of DNA or at a first approximation about 0.1% of the human X chromosome. It is divided into 26 exons and 25 introns (Fig. 1). The coding DNA (exon length) is 9 kb, of which 7053 nucleotides (nts) code for the 2351 amino acids and the rest are 5' and 3' untranslated sequences. The complete nucleotide sequence of the coding regions, the promoter elements, the intron–exon boundaries, and the deduced amino acid sequence have been determined (Git-

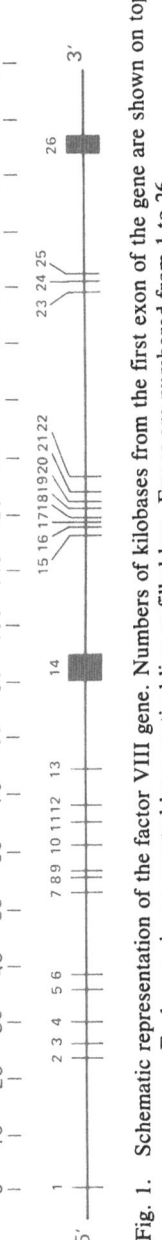

Fig. 1.   Schematic representation of the factor VIII gene. Numbers of kilobases from the first exon of the gene are shown on top. Each exon is represented by a vertical line or filled box. Exons are numbered from 1 to 26.

schier *et al.*, 1984; Toole *et al.*, 1984; Wood *et al.*, 1984). The first 19 amino acids of the sequence comprise the secretory leader peptide of the precursor FVIII, and therefore the mature excreted polypeptide consists of 2332 amino acids. The molecular mass of the single-chain precursor FVIII is calculated to be 267,039 daltons. A striking feature of the FVIII protein is that it contains domains of internal homology (Vehar *et al.*, 1984) (Fig. 2). Computer analysis of the FVIII protein sequence revealed that there are three homologous sequences (A domain) found at amino acid positions 1–329, 380–711, and 1649–2019 of the mature polypeptide. The A domains have ~30% amino acid homology. The second and third A domains are separated by the B domain of 983 amino acids, which is extremely rich in potential asparagine-linked glycosylation sites. After the third A domain there are two C domains of 150 amino acids with ~40% homology to each other. Most of the 23 cysteine residues of the mature FVIII are located in the A and C domains. The mature polypeptide has the following structure from the amino terminus to the carboxyl terminus: A_1-A_2-B-A_3-C_1-C_2. It is of interest that the A domains show striking homology (about 30%) with the three domains of the copper-binding plasma protein ceruloplasmin, and that the B domain is encoded by the unusually long (3106 nt) exon 14.

Factor VIII (VIII:C) circulates in the plasma in conjunction with von Willebrand factor, a large polymer of a polypeptide encoded by an autosomal gene on human chromosome 12 (Hoyer, 1981; Ginsburg *et al.*, 1985). Factor VIII isolated from plasma is usually degraded because it suffers proteolytic cleavages during its activation (Rotblat *et al.*, 1985). Detailed discussion of the FVIII protein biochemistry is beyond the scope of this chapter, but it is thought that a 90,000 dalton polypeptide, which contains the first two A domains (N-terminus), and an 80,000-dalton polypeptide, which contains the third A and both C domains (C-terminus), and which result after thrombin cleavage, are necessary for the "activated" form of factor VIII (VIII:Ca). Furthermore, the large B domain is cleaved off and is not required for the "activated" factor VIII (Vehar *et al.*, 1984).

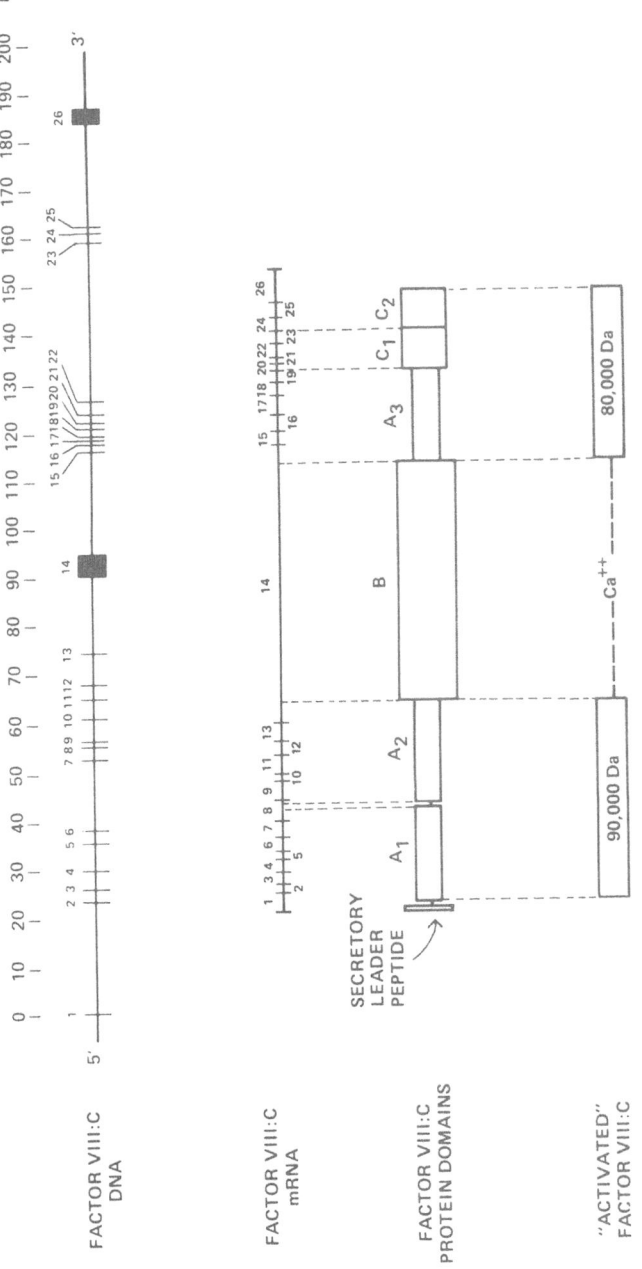

Fig. 2. Schematic representation of factor VIII gene, mRNA, protein domains, and "activated" form. The arrangement of secretory leader peptide, A_1, A_2, A_3, B, C_1, and C_2 domains of the factor VIII protein is shown and the relationship with the coding sequences of the mRNA is depicted. The "activated" form of factor VIII consists of two polypeptide chains: a heavy, 90-kilodalton (kDa) chain and a light, 80-kDa chain, which contain A_1A_2 and $A_3C_1C_2$ domains, respectively.

TABLE I. Mutations in Factor VIII Gene

Investigator[a]	Patients	Deletions	Point mutations[a]
J. Gitschier and R. Lawn	120	2	3
S. Antonarakis and H. Kazazian	80	6	6
N. Din	30	1	0
G. Camerino	45	1	0
M. Pirastu	30	1	1
D. Lillicrap	15	1	0
Total	320	12	10

[a] For references, see under specific mutations in Table II.

Mutations in the Factor VIII Gene in Hemophilia A

Hemophilia A patients can be divided according to clinical severity into moderate, mild, and severe, and this relates closely to the biological clotting factor VIII activity. In the great majority of patients, the biological activity closely parallels the amount of factor VIII protein in plasma as measured by immunological methods (Lazarchick and Hoyer, 1978). In addition, some 6–12% of patients with hemophilia A develop antibodies against factor VIII (inhibitor patients) after therapy with exogenous factor VIII (Brinkhous et al., 1972; Gill, 1984). Almost all patients with inhibitors to factor VIII have no detectable factor VIII in their plasma.

In the last year several groups of investigators from the United States (The Johns Hopkins University School of Medicine and Genentech), Canada, and Europe have examined the DNA of more than 300 patients with hemophilia A and found the molecular defect in 24 patients. Deletions of the factor VIII gene, as well as single nucleotide changes, have been found as a cause of hemophilia A (Table I). These mutations provided us with new insights into the pathogenesis of hemophilia A, the existence of "hotspots" for mutation, and the phenomenon that a considerable number of mutations to hemophilia A occur de novo.

Deletions of the Factor VIII Gene

The following deletions of the factor VIII gene have been found (Fig. 3 and Table II):

1. Deletion of about 60 kb that eliminates exons 11–19 of the factor VIII gene. The proband in this family of northern European extraction developed inhibitors to factor VIII and had severe hemophilia A with no detectable factor VIII levels (Antonarakis et al., 1985a).

2. Deletion of about 39 kb that eliminates exons 23–25. The proband had severe hemophilia A and developed inhibitors to FVIII (Gitschier et al., 1985c).

3. Deletion of about 22 kb that eliminates exon 26. The proband had severe hemophilia A, but no antibodies against factor VIII (Gitschier et al., 1985c).

4. Deletion of about 7 kb that eliminates exon 6 of the factor VIII gene. The proband, of Greek origin, had severe hemophilia A and never developed inhibitors (Youssoufian et al., 1987).

5. Deletion of about 2.5 kb that eliminates the 5′ part of exon 14 of the factor VIII gene. The proband had severe hemophilia, and no antibodies against factor VIII have been found (Youssoufian et al., 1987a).

6. Deletion of at least 3.4 kb that eliminates exons 24 and 25 of the factor VIII gene. The proband had severe hemophilia A and was inhibitor-negative. Restriction analysis of DNA from members of this family and DNA polymorphism analysis showed that the mutation occurred de novo in an X chromosome of the maternal grandmother's germ cells (Youssoufian et al., 1987).

7. Deletion of at least 9.5 kb that eliminates exons 23–25 of the factor VIII gene. The proband had severe hemophilia A and was inhibitor-negative. This deletion is different from the one described in case 2, since the 5′ end point is not the same as in case 2 (Youssoufian et al., 1986a).

8. Deletion of about 6 kb that eliminates exon 22 of the factor VIII gene. The proband had a moderately severe form of hemophilia A, with factor VIII levels of 2–5 U/dl and no inhibitors to factor

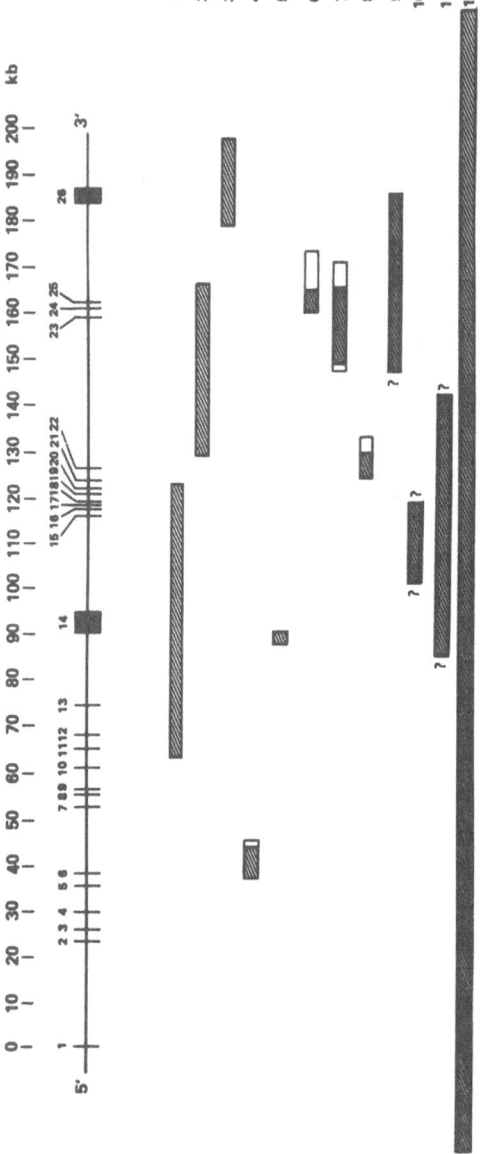

Fig. 3. Deletions of the factor VIII gene in hemophilia A. The factor VIII gene is shown on top. Each horizontal bar represents a different deletion within the factor VIII gene. Open bars at the ends of some deletions denote the uncertainty of the extent of the deletion. A question mark denotes that the extent of the deletion is unknown. The number to the right of each deletion corresponds to the number in the text. For references, see text.

TABLE II. Mutations in the Factor VIII Gene

Mutation	Severity of hemophilia A	Inhibitors to factor VIII	Reference	Number in text
Deletions:				
Deletion ~60 kb, exons 11–19	Severe	Yes	Antonarakis et al. (1985a)	1
Deletion ~39 kb, exons 23–25	Severe	Yes	Gitschier et al. (1985c)	2
Deletion ~22 kb, exon 26	Severe	No	Gitschier et al. (1985c)	3
Deletion ~7 kb, exon 6	Severe	No	Youssoufian et al. (1987)	4
Deletion ~2.5 kb, exon 14	Severe	No	Youssoufian et al. (1987)	5
Deletion >3.4 kb, exons 24–25	Severe	No	Youssoufian et al. (1987)	6
Deletion >9.5 kb, exons 23–25	Severe	No	Youssoufian et al. (1987)	7
Deletion 6 kb, exon 22	Moderate	No	Youssoufian et al. (1987)	8
Deletion exons 23–26	Severe	Yes	Din et al. (1986)	9
Deletion ~15 kb, exons 15–18	Severe	Yes	Camerino et al. (1986)	10
Deletion exons 14–22	Severe	Yes	D. Lillicrap (personal communication, 1986)	11
Deletion >210 kb, exons 1–26	Severe	No	Casarino et al. (1986)	12
Point mutations:				
CGA–TGA, nonsense codon 1960, exon 18	Severe	Yes	Antonarakis et al. (1985a)	1
CGA–TGA, nonsense codon 2326, exon 26	Severe	No	Gitschier et al. (1985c)	2
CGA–CAA, Arg–Gln, codon 2326, exon 26	Mild	No	Gitschier et al. (1986)	3
CGA–TGA, nonsense codon 2135, exon 22	Severe	No	Youssoufian et al. (1986a)	4
CGA–TGA, nonsense codon 2228, exon 24	Severe	Yes	Gitschier et al. (1985c)	5
CGA–TGA nonsense codon 2166, exon 23	Severe	Yes	H. Youssoufian et al. (1988)	6

VIII. One possible explanation of the moderate clinical phenotype is the fact that the elimination of exon 22, which encodes for 52 amino acids of the C_1 domain, leaves an in-frame junction between exons 21 and 23, and therefore the translation machinery will "read" correctly the remaining part of the molecule (Youssoufian *et al.*, 1987).

9. Deletion of exons 23–25 and part of 26 in a patient with severe hemophilia A and inhibitors to factor VIII (Din *et al.*, 1986).

10. Deletion of about 15 kb that eliminates exons 15–18 in a patient with severe hemophilia A and inhibitors to factor VIII (Camerino *et al.*, 1986).

11. Deletion of exons 14–22 (preliminary analysis) in a patient with severe hemophilia A and inhibitors to factor VIII (D. Lillicrap, personal communication, Milan, 1986).

12. Deletion of at least 210 kb that eliminates the entire factor VIII gene. The 3' end of the deletion was localized to about 30 kb 3' to the poly A site of the factor VIII gene. The mutation occurred *de novo* in the maternal germ cells. The proband had severe hemophilia and did not develop inhibitors to factor VIII (Casarino *et al.*, 1986).

In summary, all but one of the partial factor VIII gene deletions described to date are associated with severe hemophilia A. Five of 12 deletions were associated with the presence of antibodies against factor VIII (cases 1, 2, and 9–11). No definitive conclusions can be drawn concerning the association of inhibitor formation and the size and position of the deletion. More data are necessary to address this question. Finally, it is of interest that 12 of 320 patients (3.75%) with hemophilia A examined have sizable deletions within the factor VIII gene, which can be recognized by simple restriction analysis.

Single-Nucleotide Mutations within the Factor VIII Gene

Although the gene for factor VIII is enormous and it seemed unlikely that single-nucleotide changes would be identified using restriction analysis, the following mutations have been identified and are shown in Fig. 4 and Table II:

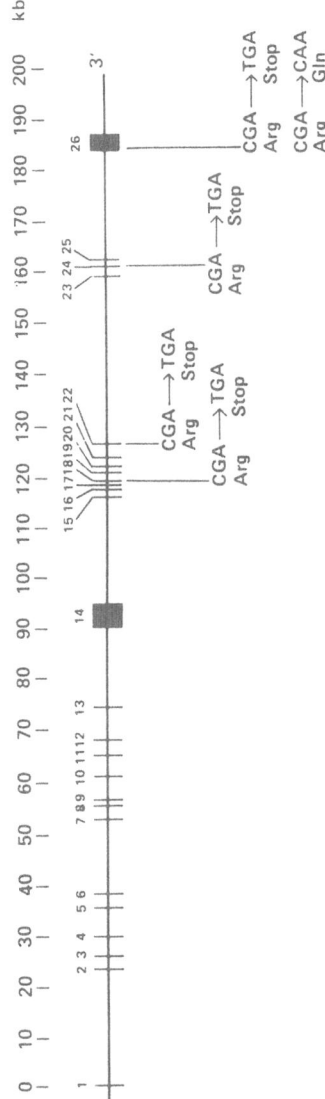

Fig. 4.   Single-nucleotide mutations within the factor VIII gene. The nucleotide changes and the amino acid changes are shown. Arg: arginine; Gln: glutamine; stop: nonsense codon.

1. CGA–TGA in codon 1960, exon 18 of the factor VIII gene. The single-nucleotide C–T substitution converts the codon for arginine to a nonsense codon and translation stops prematurely (Antonarakis *et al.*, 1985*a*). This mutation occurs in the recognition sequence of restriction endonuclease *Taq*I and was characterized by oligonucleotide hybridization experiments using both normal and mutant synthetic oligonucleotides as probes. This mutation was found in two families. One was of British extraction and the other was a Greek family. In the latter family it was shown that the mutation occurred *de novo* in the maternal grandfather's germ cells (Youssoufian *et al.*, 1987). (This individual was 32 years old when his carrier daughter was conceived.) Nonpaternity was excluded at the 10^{-6} level. This was the first convincing and unequivocal report of independent origins of the same mutation in hemophilia A. The probands from both families had developed antibodies (inhibitors) against factor VIII, although in the Greek family there were affected members without inhibitors. All patients had severe hemophilia A with no detectable factor VIII.

2. CGA–TGA in codon 2326, exon 26 of the factor VIII gene. The single-nucleotide C–T substitution converts the codon for arginine to a nonsense codon, only 26 amino acids before the normal termination site (Gitschier *et al.*, 1985*c*). This mutation also occurs in a *Taq*I recognition sequence and was characterized by cloning and sequencing of the abnormal factor VIII gene. The proband had severe hemophilia A and did not develop inhibitors to factor VIII. This mutation suggests that the last 26 amino acids of the mature factor VIII polypeptide are crucial for its biological activity.

3. CGA–CAA in codon 2326, exon 26 of the factor VIII gene. The single-nucleotide change G–A converts the codon for arginine to a codon for glutamine (Gitschier *et al.*, 1986). It is noteworthy that this missense mutation occurred in the same codon as the previous one and within the recognition sequence of the same *Taq*I site. The proband's phenotype is strikingly different from that of the patient with the nonsense codon. In the Arg–Gln change the hemophilia A is mild, with 10% normal factor VIII activity and no inhibitors to factor VIII. The mutation was characterized by oligonucleotide hybridization.

4. CGA–TGA in codon 2135, exon 22 of the factor VIII gene. The single-nucleotide change C–T converts the codon for arginine to a nonsense codon, which results in a premature termination of translation (Youssoufian *et al.*, 1986). The mutation also occurs in the recognition sequence of *Taq*I and was characterized by oligonucleotide hybridization. The mutation was found in two families of northern European extraction unrelated to each other. In one of these families it was shown that the mutation occurred *de novo* in the maternal grandfather's germ cells, and this individual was 34 years old when his carrier daughter was conceived. This is another example of the recurrent origin of the same mutation. The affected individuals from both families had severe hemophilia A with no detectable factor VIII activity and no inhibitors to factor VIII.

5. CGA–TGA in codon 2228, exon 24 of the factor VIII gene. The single-nucleotide change C–T also produces an Arg-stop codon and premature termination of translation (Gitschier *et al.*, 1985c). The mutation, which also occurs in a *Taq*I recognition site, was characterized by cloning and sequencing of the abnormal gene. The proband had severe hemophilia and high titers of inhibitors to factor VIII. Restriction analysis in different family members suggested that the patient's mother was not a carrier of the mutation and therefore it occurred *de novo* in a maternal germ cell.

6. CGA–TGA in codon 2166, exon 23 of the factor VIII gene. The single nucleotide change C–T converts for arginine to a nonsense codon, which results in a premature termination of translation. The mutation also occurs in the recognition sequence of *Taq*I and is characterized by oligonucleotide hybridization. Hemophilia A was severe in this family and inhibitors to factor VIII were observed (Youssoufian *et al.*, 1988).

In summary, five different single-nucleotide substitutions were found in the factor VIII gene that produced hemophilia A in seven pedigrees. The mutations arose *de novo* in three of these seven families. All of these mutations occurred in *Taq*I recognition sites and affect CpG dinucleotides. The CpG dinucleotides are thought to be "hotspots" for mutation because C can be methylated at the 5 position of the pyrimidine ring and subsequently spontaneously deaminated to thymine (T). This accounts for CG–TG and CG–CA mutations. That CpG dinucleotides are "hotspots" for mutations is also supported by the fact that a considerable number of DNA polymorphic sites are in restriction endonuclease recognition sequences that contain CpG (*Taq*I and *Msp*I, for example) (Barker *et al.*, 1984). Factor VIII gene contains seven *Taq*I sites in its coding region, five of which have CGA as a codon for arginine. Mutations have been observed in four of these five *Taq*I sites (exons 18, 22, 24, 26) and another is suspected in the fifth site in exon 23 (case 6 of point mutations). The data collected to date support the Haldane hypothesis that in about one-third of hemophiliacs there is a *de novo* mutation. It is of interest that there are two examples (cases 2 and 4) in which the same mutation was observed in less than 200 defective factor VIII genes, and one can calculate that up to 10,000 recurrences of the same exact mutation may have occurred in man in the last 2000 years.

DNA Polymorphisms in the Factor VIII Gene

Since each family with hemophilia A usually has a different mutation in the factor VIII gene, it is almost impossible to detect directly the molecular defect using restriction endonuclease and prenatal diagnosis. On the other hand, indirect detection of the abnormal factor VIII gene (regardless of the nature of the abnormality) can be achieved using as markers DNA polymorphisms within or adjacent to the factor VIII gene. In the past year there has been a considerable effort to identify DNA polymorphisms within the factor VIII gene, but the yield has been relatively poor. The following high-frequency polymorphic sites within the factor VIII gene have been identified (Fig. 5).

1. *Bcl*I site within intron 18 of the factor VIII gene comprising a two-allele system with DNA fragment sizes 1.2 and 0.9 kb (Gitschier *et al.*, 1985c). The frequency of the presence of the polymorphic site was about 50% in Mediterraneans, 60% in northern Europeans, 70% in Asiatic Indians, and 20% in American blacks (Gitschier *et al.*, 1985c; Antonarakis *et al.*, 1985a). This site is an excellent marker for carrier detection and prenatal diagnosis (An-

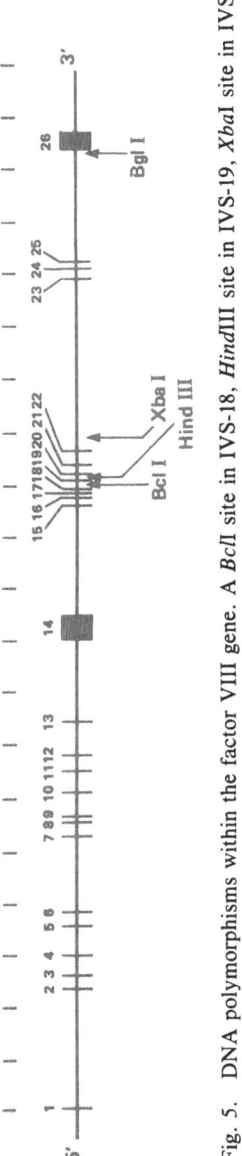

Fig. 5. DNA polymorphisms within the factor VIII gene. A *BcI*I site in IVS-18, *Hind*III site in IVS-19, *Xba*I site in IVS-22, and *Bgl*I site at the 3' end of IVS-25 are depicted.

tonarakis *et al.*, 1985*b*; Gitschier *et al.*, 1985*b*; Din *et al.*, 1985) because about 50% of Caucasian women are heterozygotes for this polymorphic site.

2. *Bgl*I site in intron 25 just 2 kb 5' of exon 26 of the factor VIII gene, comprising a two-allele system with DNA fragment sizes of 5 and 20 kb. The frequency of the presence of the *Bgl*I polymorphic site is about 90% in Caucasians and 75% in American blacks (Antonarakis *et al.*, 1985*a*). It is therefore a relatively good marker for carrier detection and prenatal diagnosis in the American black population. There is a low level of linkage disequilibrium between the *Bcl*I and *Bgl*I sites, and therefore, combined use of both sites does not dramatically increase the yield of informative (heterozygous females for at least one marker) pedigrees. In fact, about 60–70% of the families who seek prenatal diagnosis and/or carrier detection of hemophilia A in the United States were informative for *Bgl*I and/or *Bcl*I polymorphic sites (Phillips *et al.*, 1985).

3. *Xba*I site in intron 22 of the factor VIII gene. This is a recently reported DNA polymorphic site from Genentech (Wion *et al.*, 1986). The allelic DNA fragments are 6.2 and 1.4 kb. The frequency of the presence of this polymorphic site in a mixed population from San Francisco was about 60%. In addition, there is some linkage disequilibrium, but not a high degree, with the *Bcl*I polymorphic site, and therefore about 25% of females who are homozygous for the *Bcl*I site are heterozygous for the *Xba*I polymorphic site.

4. *Hind*III site in intron 19 of the factor VIII gene, recently reported (Ahrens *et al.*, 1987). The allelic fragments are 2.6 and 2.7 kb. The frequency of the presence of this polymorphic site in Caucasians is 0.30. There is a high degree of linkage disequilibrium between the *Bcl*I site (intron 18) and this *Hind*III site. Therefore, the clinical usefulness of the *Hind*III site is very limited.

If one uses these polymorphic sites as markers for the normal and the abnormal factor VIII alleles in families, the error in carrier detection and/or prenatal diagnosis is negligible because the recombination rate between a given marker and the actual site of mutation will be extremely low.

Other DNA polymorphic markers have been described that are

very tightly linked with the factor VIII gene and the hemophilia A phenotype. These markers are as follows:

1. DNA polymorphisms *Taq*I and *Msp*I associated with probe ST14 or DXS52. This is an extremely useful and informative polymorphic system in which several alleles from the same locus can be recognized (Oberle *et al.*, 1985*a,b*). The genetic distance between DXS52 and factor VIII was initially reported to be 0 cM because no recombinants were found between the marker and either the hemophilia phenotype or the factor VIII gene. Recently, as part of our analyses for carrier detection and prenatal diagnosis, we have identified two potential recombinants between DXS52 and the factor VIII locus. The possibility of nonpaternity has not been excluded with a high level of significance in these families. After the initial reports of tight linkage between DXS52 and factor VIII gene, several investigators observed six recombinants in 133 chances for recombination (I. Peake, personal communication, Milan, 1986; Driscoll *et al.*, 1986). A conservative view might be that there is about 3–5% recombinational distance between DXS52 and factor VIII and therefore an unavoidable 3–5% error in the DNA diagnosis of the presence or absence of the mutant allele in a given family.

2. *Bgl*II site adjacent to DNA probe DX13 or DXS15. This latter probe also maps to the same chromosomal band as DXS52 and factor VIII and is tightly linked with factor VIII (Harper *et al.*, 1984). However, several recombinants have been recognized between these two markers, and the recombination distance might well be on the order of 2–5%. From the recombinant that we recently observed in a family that was informative for all three markers DXS15, DXS52, and factor VIII the crossing-over occurred between DXS15 and factor VIII, between DXS52 and factor VIII, but not between DXS15 and DXS52. If one crossover was responsible for these data, then DXS15 and DXS52 most likely were on the same side of factor VIII and therefore they are not flanking DNA markers. It is important to reemphasize the error rate in gene diagnosis using DXS15 as marker for the factor VIII gene. The use of both intragenic factor VIII markers and DXS15 and DXS52 will provide mutant factor VIII gene diagnosis in almost all affected pedigrees with a positive family

history and family members available for study and linkage analysis (Janco *et al.*, 1986).

HEMOPHILIA B. FACTOR IX GENE

Cloning and Characterization of Factor IX Gene

By 1979 the entire amino acid sequence of the bovine factor IX was known (Katayama *et al.*, 1979). Three groups, Brownlee and co-workers, Davie and co-workers, and Transgene (a biotechnology company), used synthetic oligonucleotide probe mixtures for several regions of bovine factor IX to isolate successfully the bovine cDNA and subsequently to clone and characterize the human factor IX gene (Choo *et al.*, 1982; Kurachi and Davie, 1982; Jaye *et al.*, 1983). This gene is 34 kb long and is divided into eight exons and seven intervening sequences (Fig. 6) and includes sequences for a 46-amino acid precursor polypeptide (Anson *et al.*, 1984). The complete nucleotide sequence of the entire gene including the coding regions, the promoter elements, and the introns and the corresponding amino acid sequence has been established (Yoshitake *et al.*, 1985). Factor IX is synthesized in the liver as a single-chain precursor and then is processed during its secretion into the bloodstream. The first 46 amino acids at the N-terminus (prepro leader sequence) are removed during biosynthesis by signal peptidase and a processing protease. The mature protein contains 415 amino acids and consists of the following domains: the first is called Gla domain (residues 1–145) and is homologous with human epidermal growth factor (EGF). The second domain (residues 146–180) is called the activation peptide and is released from factor IX during its conversion to factor IXa. The third domain (residues 181–415) is the serine protease or catalytic domain and includes the active site that participates in catalysis (Kurachi *et al.*, 1982). Factor IX is also posttranslationally modified by hydroxylation of the β-carbon of aspartic acid at reside 64 of the mature protein, and by γ-carboxylation of the most N-terminal 12 glutamic acid residues. Both modifications are essential for activity. Comparison of the factor IX gene and other members of the

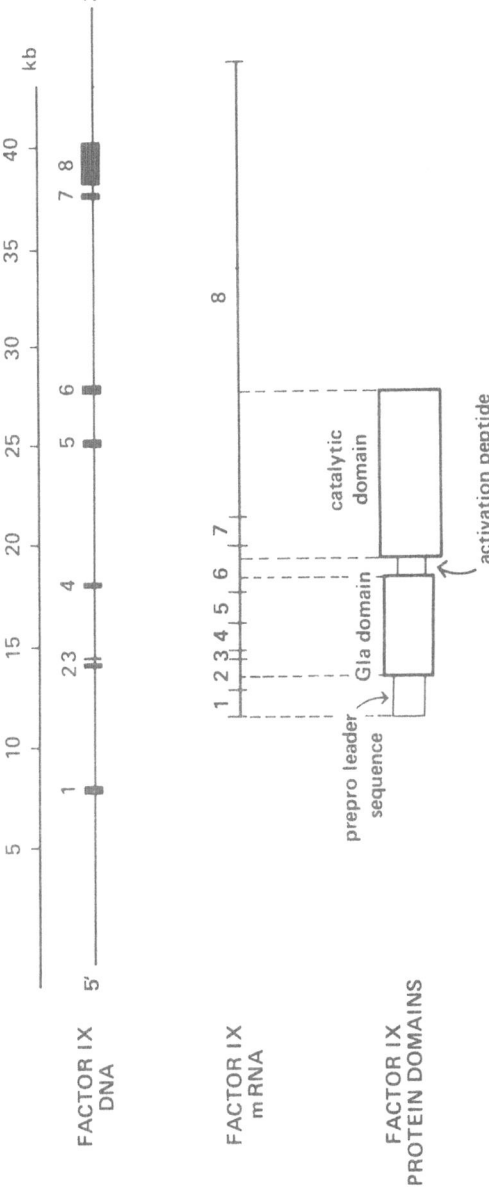

Fig. 6.   Schematic representation of factor IX gene, its corresponding mRNA, and the factor IX protein domains. A kilobase scale is shown on top. The gene has eight exons (represented as filled bars). The protein domains and their corresponding exons are also depicted.

serine protease superfamily reveals interesting evolutionary examples of exon shuffling and intron insertion and loss.

Mutations in the Factor IX Gene in Hemophilia B

As with factor VIII deficiency, hemophilia B is heterogeneous and patients can be subdivided into three classes: those with immunologically detectable but reduced levels of factor IX (crm^+R), those with no detectable factor IX (crm^-), and those with normal concentrations of factor IX antigen in their plasma (crm^+). It is expected that crm^+ patients might have missense mutations in coding regions, splicing mutations, or transcription mutations that result in reduced amounts of factor IX. The crm^- group of patients might have frameshift and missense mutations resulting in unstable protein products, nonsense mutations, severe splice junction defects, severe promoter mutations, and gene deletions. A group of crm^- patients develop "inhibitors" or anti-factor IX antibodies in their plasma in response to replacement therapy.

Deletions of the Factor IX Gene

The following deletions including part or the entire factor IX gene have been described (Fig. 7 and Table III):

1–3. Three deletions in the factor IX gene were reported by Giannelli et al. (1983). The extent of each deletion was not fully characterized, but all are different. Two are complete gene deletions. The third eliminates a segment of approximately 30 kb containing exons 6–8 of the factor IX gene (F. Giannelli, personal communication, London, 1986). The patients with these deletions had severe hemophilia B and developed inhibitors to factor IX.

4. Deletion of 10 ± 0.3 kb, which eliminates exons 5 and 6. The proband had severe hemophilia B and did not have inhibitors to factor IX (Chen et al., 1985).

5. Deletion of approximately 33 kb of the factor IX gene in an Italian patient. The deletion extends from about 7.5 kb 5′ to the first exon to approximately 125 nts within the last exon (exon 8). The

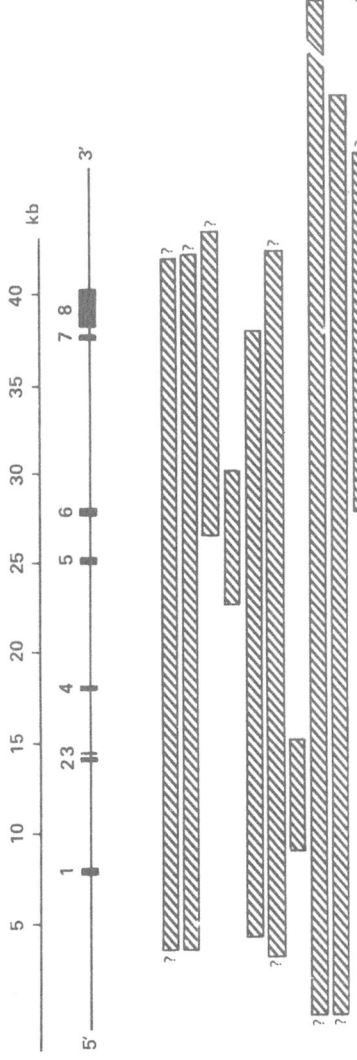

Fig. 7. Deletions of the factor IX gene in hemophilia B. Each horizontal bar represents a different deletion. A question mark denotes that the extent of the deletion is unknown. The number to the right of each deletion corresponds to the number in the text. For references, see text.

TABLE III. Mutation in the Factor IX Gene

Mutation	Severity of hemophilia B	Inhibitors to factor IX	Reference	Number in text
Deletions:				
Deletion exons 1–8, unknown size	Severe	Yes	Giannelli et al. (1983)	1
Deletion exons 1–8, unknown size	Severe	Yes	Giannelli et al. (1983)	2
Deletion exons 6–8	Severe	Yes	Giannelli et al. (1983)	3
Deletion ~10 kb, exons 5–6	Severe	No	Chen et al. (1985)	4
Deletion ~33 kb, exons 1–8	Severe	Yes	Hassan et al. (1985)	5
Deletion large, unknown size	Severe	Yes	Bernardi et al. (1985)	6
Deletion 7–9 kb, exons 2–3	Severe	Yes	M. Ludwig et al. (personal communication, 1986)	7
Deletion >115 kb, exons 1–8	Severe	Yes	Peake et al. (1984), Peake and Matthews (1986)	8
Deletion >110 kb, exons 1–8	Severe	Yes	Peake and Matthews (1986)	9
Deletion exons 7–8	Severe	Yes	Peake and Matthews (1986)	10
Point mutations:				
Factor IX Chapel Hill Arg–His, CGT–CAT, codon 145, exon 6	Mild	No	Noyes et al. (1983)	1
Factor IX Alabama Asp–Gly, GAT–GGT, codon 47, exon 3	Mild	No	Davis et al. (1984)	2
CGG–CAG, Arg–Gln, codon −4, exon 2	Mild	No	Bentley et al. (1986)	3
GT–TT, IVS-6 nt 1	Severe	No	Rees et al. (1985)	4
GT–GG, IVS-3 nt 2	Severe	No	Winship et al. (1984)	5

proband had severe hemophilia B and developed inhibitors to factor IX (Hassan *et al.*, 1985).

6. Large deletion of the factor IX gene in an Italian patient with severe hemophilia B and inhibitors to factor IX (Bernardi *et al.*, 1985).

7. Deletion of approximately 7–9 kb that eliminates exons 2 and 3 of the factor IX gene. The proband had severe crm⁻ hemophilia B and developed inhibitors to factor IX (M. Ludwig and K. Olek, personal communication, Milan, 1986).

8. Deletion of at least 115 kb that eliminates the entire factor IX gene. The proband had severe hemophilia B and developed inhibitors to factor IX (Peake *et al.*, 1984; Peake and Matthews, 1986).

9. Deletion of at least 110 kb that eliminates the entire factor IX gene. The proband had severe hemophilia B and developed inhibitors to factor IX (Peake and Matthews, 1986).

10. Deletion of exons 7–8 of the factor IX gene in a patient with severe hemophilia B and inhibitors to factor IX (Peake and Matthews, 1986). The deletion starts within 800 base pairs of the 3′ end of exon 6 and ends less than 25 kb 3′ to exon 8.

In the case of hemophilia B, there is a strong correlation between inhibitors to factor IX and the presence of partial or complete gene deletions. In the 15 patients with hemophilia B and inhibitors to factor IX examined to date, 5 complete and 4 partial factor IX gene deletions have been found, while in 6 such patients no gross deletions or rearrangement of the factor IX gene was observed (I. R. Peake, personal communication, Milan, 1986). This is in contrast to the deletions found in the factor VIII gene, in which many of the deletions were not associated with inhibitors to factor VIII.

Single-Nucleotide Mutations within the Factor IX Gene

The following single-nucleotide mutations that cause hemophilia B have been identified within the factor IX gene (Fig. 8 and Table III):

1. Factor IX Chapel Hill. This is an abnormal factor IX from a patient with CRM⁺ antigen. The abnormality has been charac-

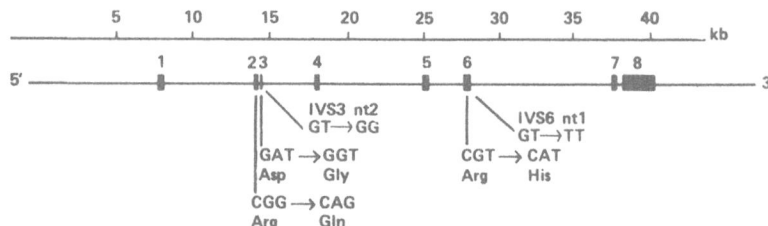

Fig. 8. Single-nucleotide mutations within the factor IX gene. The nucleotide changes and the amino acid changes are shown. Asp: asparagine; Arg: arginine; Gln: glutamine; His: histidine.

terized by amino acid sequencing. There is an Arg–His change at amino acid residue 145 of the mature factor IX polypeptide (Noyes et al., 1983). The deduced nucleotide mutation presumably is CGT–CAT at the appropriate codon in exon 6. The mutation results in failure to cleave at one of the sites of activation and therefore reduces activity of the factor IX protein.

2. Factor IX Alabama. This is also an abnormal factor IX molecule from a patient with CRM$^+$ antigen. The abnormality is the replacement of Asp by Gly at amino acid residue 47 (exon 3) of the mature factor IX polypeptide (Davis et al., 1984). The deduced nucleotide mutation presumably is GAT–GGT at the appropriate codon in exon 3. The mutation occurs in the epidermal growth factor homology region of the factor IX polypeptide.

3. CGG–CAG at codon −4, exon 2 of the factor IX gene (nucleotide 6365). The mutation converts Arg–Gln and alters a HaeIII restriction site (Bentley et al., 1986). The abnormal factor IX was termed Oxford 3 and occurs in a patient with hemophilia B who had 89% factor IX antigen and <0.5% clotting activity. The molecular weight of the "mature" factor IX polypeptide was slightly higher than normal. The Arg–Gln change apparently prevents propeptide processing, which results in an abnormally long polypeptide with an N-terminal extension of 18 amino acids accumulating in the plasma. The proband had crm$^+$ hemophilia B.

4. GT–TT in the first nucleotide of IVS-6 (donor splicing site) of the factor IX gene (Rees et al., 1985). The proband had severe crm$^-$ hemophilia B. This mutation is reminiscent of a β^0-thalassemia

mutation at the same nucleotide of IVS-1 of the β-globin gene and underlines the importance of the invariant GT dinucleotide in the donor splice site.

5. GT–GG in the second nucleotide of IVS-3 (donor splicing site) of the factor IX gene (Winship *et al.*, cited in Brownlee, 1986). The proband also had severe crm⁻ hemophilia B, because no normal RNA splicing occurs when the second invariant nucleotide of the donor consensus splicing sequence is mutated. No inhibitors have been detected in any of the patients with the point mutations described.

It is noteworthy that two of these mutations occur in CG dinucleotides as a result of a probable methylation–deamination CG–TG or CG–CA mutation, as discussed in the factor VIII section.

DNA Polymorphisms in the Factor IX Gene

For the reasons discussed under the factor VIII gene, it is extremely important to recognize the mutant factor IX gene indirectly, regardless of the exact molecular defect. This can be accomplished with the use of DNA polymorphic sites within the factor IX gene. The following polymorphic sites have been described (Fig. 9).

1. *Taq*I site in IVS-4 of the factor IX gene. The allelic fragments are 1.3 and 1.8 kb. The frequency of the presence of this site is about

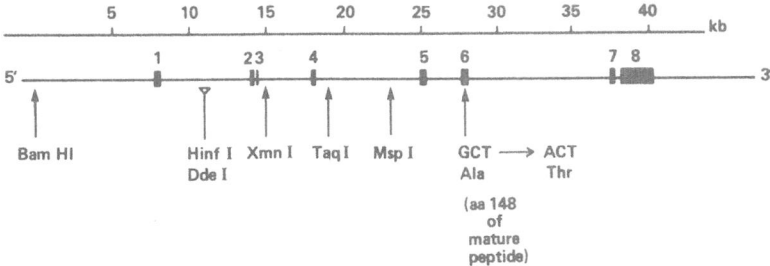

Fig. 9. DNA polymorphisms within the factor IX gene. *Bam*HI, *Xmn*I, *Taq*I, and *Msp*I are single-nucleotide change polymorphisms, as is the GCT to ACT mutation in exon 6, which changes alanine to threonine in the mature protein. The *Hinf*I or *Dde*I polymorphism is due to a 50-nucleotide insertion in IVS-1 of the factor IX gene.

30% in Caucasians, and therefore about 40% of females are heterozygotes for this site (Giannelli *et al.*, 1984; Grunebaum *et al.*, 1984).

2. *Msp*I site in IVS-4 of the factor IX gene. The allelic fragment
sizes are 2.4 and 5.8 kb and the frequency of the presence of this
site is about 80% in Caucasians (Camerino *et al.*, 1985).

3. *Xmn*I site in IVS-3 of the factor IX gene. The allelic fragment
sizes are 11.5 kb (when the site is absent) and 6.5 and 5.0 kb (when
the site is present); the frequency of the presence of the site is about
30% in the British population (Winship *et al.*, 1984).

4. DNA polymorphism due to an insertion of 50 nucleotides in
IVS-1 of the factor IX gene. The presence of these 50 nts results in
a 1.75-kb fragment after cleavage of DNA with *Dde*I or a 0.80-kb
fragment after cleavage with *Hinf*I and hybridization with the appropriate probe. The absence of the 50 nts results in a 1.70- or 0.75-
kb fragment using these enzymes, respectively. The presence of
these 50 nts has a frequency of 25% of the factor IX alleles in British
subjects (Winship *et al.*, 1984).

5. G–A polymorphism in residue 609 of mRNA of the factor
IX gene, which produces an Ala–Thr polymorphism in the amino
acid sequence (amino acid 148 of the mature polypeptide) (Yoshitake
et al., 1985). This polymorphic site can be best recognized by oligonucleotide hybridization (G. Brownlee, personal communication,
Milan, 1986).

6. *Bam*HI polymorphic site 5′ to the factor IX gene (Hay *et al.*,
1986; B. Migeon, personal communication, Baltimore, 1986).

There is considerable linkage disequilibrium between the *Taq*I
and *Xmn*I sites and the 50-nt insertion polymorphism. Using the
above-mentioned sites it is possible to perform carrier detection and
prenatal diagnosis in 70% of Caucasian families with hemophilia B.
The accuracy of the detection of the mutant gene is very high (prac-
tically 100%) because the polymorphic sites are intragenic and negligible recombination occurs between the polymorphic site and the
site of mutation in one generation in a family. More DNA polymorphic markers are needed to provide diagnosis of the defective
allele in almost all families with hemophilia B with a positive family
history, in whom appropriate family linkage studies can be performed, and in which an afffected individual is available for study.

X-CHROMOSOME MAPPING OF FACTOR VIII
AND IX GENES

It has been well known that both hemophilia A and B are X-linked disorders (McKusick, 1962). The cloning of factor IX and factor VIII genes and the discovery of DNA polymorphic markers within or closely linked to these genes enabled the improvement of the accuracy of the genetic map of the X chromosome in the area Xq27–qter where these genes lie. *In situ* hybridization in early metaphase chromosomes using factor IX molecular probes had established the location of factor IX at Xq27 (more precisely, Xq27.1) (Boyd *et al.*, 1984; Purrello *et al.*, 1985; Mattei *et al.*, 1985). The hemophilia A locus (factor VIII) is known to be closely linked with the genes for glucose-6-phosphate dehydrogenase (G6PD), color-blindness, and adrenoleukodystrophy (ALD) [summarized in Keats (1983)]. It has been shown by *in situ* hybridization and the use of somatic cell hybrids that factor VIII maps to Xq28 (Purello *et al.*, 1985). Several groups of investigators have estimated the genetic recombination distances between factor IX, factor VIII, and the fragile X site (FRAXA), which maps in Xq27 between the two clotting factor genes [Goodfellow *et al.* (1985) for review]. The map distance between factor IX and factor VIII genes was estimated in several studies to be about 30 cM (Gitschier *et al.*, 1985*a*; Drayna and White, 1985; Oberle *et al.*, 1986). The map distance between factor IX and the fragile Xq27 site was estimated to be $\theta = 0.125$ and that between the fragile Xq27 site and factor VIII to be $\theta = 0.097$ (Oberle *et al.*, 1986; Brown *et al.*, 1985). The regional map of the distal long arm of chromosome X in man is shown in Fig. 10.

LESSONS FROM THE STUDY OF THE
MOLECULAR GENETICS OF HEMOPHILIA

A number of generalizations are possible from the study of factor VIII and IX genes in hemophilia. First, as expected for X-linked disorders with poor reproduction, the majority of affected families

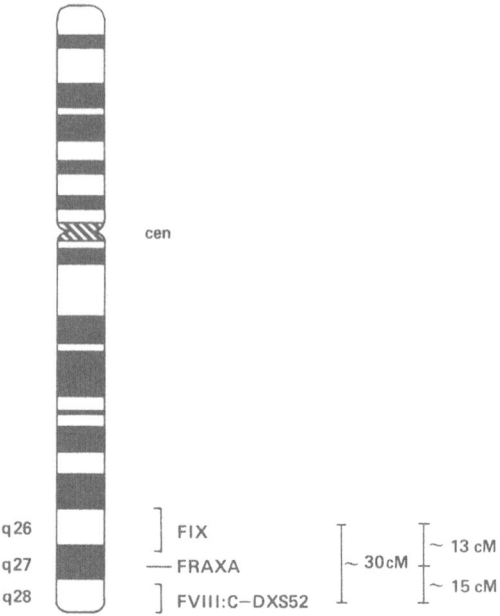

Fig. 10.   Linkage map of the distal end of the long arm of human chromosome X.
The distances in centimorgans (cM) among factor IX (FIX) gene, fragile X (FRAXA),
factor VIII (FVIII:C), and DNA marker DXS52 are depicted.

carry their own private mutant allele. Second, about 5% of the mutant alleles are deletions within the factor VIII and IX genes, in
contrast to the small number of deletions in β-thalassemia genes.
Third, a large number of point mutations have been found in CG
dinucleotides of the type CG–TG or CG–CA. These substitutions
have produced both nonsense and missense mutations. The mechanism underlying the susceptibility of CG dinucleotides is presumably methylation of cytosine (C) residues at the 5 position in the
pyrimidine ring when cytosine is located 5′ to guanine (G). Such a
methyl-C can then become spontaneously deaminated directly to
thymine (T). Thus, CG dinucleotides may represent mutation hotspots in man.

   The study of mutations in X-linked disorders will probably provide us with a relatively unbiased view of the frequency of various

types of mutations because every deleterious mutation will produce a disease phenotype in a male individual.

ACKNOWLEDGMENTS. The author thanks Dr. Haig H. Kazazian, Jr. for a most enjoyable collaboration during the factor VIII project. He also thanks Dr. R. Lawn, J. Gitschier, I. Peake, F. Giannelli, G. Brownlee, M. Pirastu, N. Din, M. Ludwig, K. Olek, D. Lillicrap, G. Camerino, L. W. Hoyer, and P. M. Mannucci for sharing unpublished data, and for helpful discussions and critical comments. He also thanks Drs. H. Youssoufian, J. Toole, J. Wozney, S. Aronis, G. Tsiftis, G. Stamatoyannopoulos, D. Fass, G. Bowie, D. Phillips, and many physicians and genetic counselors for their help in the collection of the data. He also thanks Emily Pasterfield for expert secretarial assistance. This work was supported by NIH, MOD, and JHU Institutional grants and a New Investigator Research Award.

REFERENCES

Ahrens, P., Kruse, T. A., Schwartz, M., Rasmussen, P. B., Din, N., 1986, A new *Hind* III restriction fragment length polymorphism in the hemophilia A locus, *Hum. Genet.* 76:127–128.

Anson, D. S., Choo, K. H., Rees, D. J. G., Giannelli, G., Gould, K., Huddleston, J. A., and Brownlee, G. G., 1984, Gene structure of human anti-haemophilic factor IX, *EMBO J.* 3:1053–1064.

Antonarakis, S. E., Waber, P. G., Kittur, S. D., Patel, A. S., Kazazian, H. H., Jr., Mellis, M. A., Counts, R. B., Stamatoyannapoulos, G., Bowie, E. J. W., Fass, D. N., Pittman, D. D., Wozney, J. M., and Toole, J. J., 1985a, Hemophilia A: Molecular defects and carrier detection by DNA analysis, *N. Engl. J. Med.* 313:842–848.

Antonarakis, S. E., Copeland, K. L., Carpenter, R. J., Carta, C. A., Hoyer, L. W., Caskey, C. T., Toole, J. J., and Kazazian, H. H., Jr., 1985b, Prenatal diagnosis of hemophilia A by factor VIII gene analysis, *Lancet* 1:1407–1410.

Barker, D., Schafer, M., White, R., 1984, Restriction sites containing CpG show a higher frequency of polymorphism in human DNA, *Cell* 36:131–138.

Bentley, A. K., Rees, D. J. G., Rizza, C., and Brownlee, G. G., 1986, Defective propeptide processing of blood clotting factor IX caused by mutation of arginine-4 to glutamine, *Cell* 45:343–348.

Bernardi, F., del Senno, L., Barbieri, R., Buzzoni, D., Gambari, R., Marchetti, G., Conconi, F., Panicucci, F., Positano, M., and Pitruzzello, S., 1985, Gene deletion in an Italian haemophilia B subject, *J. Med. Genet.* 22:305–307.

Boyd, Y., Buckle, V. J., Munro, E. A., Choo, K. H., Migeon, B. R., and Craig, I.

W., 1984, Assignment of the haemophilia B (factor IX) locus to the q26-qter region of the X chromosome, *Ann. Hum. Genet.* **48**:145–152.

Brinkhous, K. M., Roberts, H. R., and Weiss, A. E., 1972, Prevalence of inhibitors in hemophilia A and B, *Thromb. Diath. Haemorrh.* **51**:315–320.

Brown, W. T., Gross, A. C., Chan, C. B., and Jenkins, E. C., 1985, DNA linkage studies in the fragile X syndrome suggest genetic heterogeneity, *Hum. Genet.* **71**:11–18.

Brownlee, G. G., 1986, The molecular genetics of hemophilia A and B, *J. Cell. Sci. Suppl.* **4**:445–458.

Camerino, G., Oberle, I., Drayna, D., and Mandel, J. L., 1985, A new *Msp* I restriction fragment length polymorphism in the hemophilia B locus, *Hum. Genet.* **71**:79–81.

Camerino, G., Bardoni, B., Sampietro, M., Romano, M., Crapanzano, C., and Mannucci, D. M., 1986, Deletion of part of coagulation factor VIII in a hemophiliac with inhibitor, *Ric. Clin. Lab* **16**:227 (Abstract).

Casarino, L., Pecorara, M., Mori, P. G., Morfini, M., Mancuso, G., Scrivano, L., Molinari, A. C., Lanza, T., Giavarella, G., Loi, A., Perseu, L., Cao, A., and Pirastu, M., 1986, Molecular basis for hemophilia A in Italians, *Ric. Clin. Lab.* **16**:227 (Abstract).

Chen, S. H., Yoshitake, S., Chance, P. F., Bray, G. L., Thompson, A. R., Scott, C. R., and Kurachi, K., 1985, An intragenic gene deletion of the factor IX gene in a family with hemophilia B, *J. Clin. Invest.* **76**:2161–2164.

Choo, K. H., Gould, K. G., Rees, D. J. G., and Brownlee, G. G., 1982, Molecular cloning of the gene for human antihaemophilic factor IX, *Nature* **299**:178–180.

Davis, L. M., McGraw, R. A., Graham, J. B., Roberts, H. R., and Stafford, D. W., 1984, Identification of the genetic defect in factor IX Alabama DNA sequence reveals a GLY substitution for Asp46, *Blood* **64**:262a.

Din, N., Schwartz, M., Kruse, T. A., Vestergaard, S. R., Ahrens, P., Caput, D., Herzog, K., and Quiroga, M., 1985, Factor VIII gene specific probe for prenatal diagnosis of hemophilia A, *Lancet* **1**:1446–1447.

Din, N., Schwartz, M., Kruse, T., Vestergaard, S. R., Ahrens, P., Scheibel, E., Nordfang, O., and Ezban, M., 1986, Factor VIII gene specific probes used to study heritage and molecular defects in hemophilia A, *Ric. Clin. Lab.* **16**:182 (Abstract).

Drayna, D., and White, R., 1985, The genetic linkage map of the human X chromosome, *Science* **230**:753–758.

Driscoll, M. C., Miller, C. H., Goldberg, J. D., Aledort, L. M., Hoyer, L. W., and Golbus, M. S., 1986, Recombination between factor VIII:C gene and ST14 locus, *Lancet* **2**:279.

Fass, D. N., Knutson, G. J., and Katzmann, J. A., 1982, Monoclonal antibodies to porcine factor VIII:C and their use in the isolation of active coagulant protein, *Blood* **59**:594–600.

Giannelli, F., Choo, K. H., Rees, D. J. G., Boyd, Y., Rizza, C. R., and Brownlee, G. G., 1983, Gene deletions in patients with haemophilia B and antifactor IX antibodies, *Nature* **303**:181–182.

Giannelli, F., Choo, K. H., Winship, P. R., Anson, D. S., Rees, D. J. G., Ferrari, N., Rizza, C. R., and Brownlee, G. G., 1984, Characterization and use of an intragenic polymorphic marker for detection of carriers of haemophilia B (factor IX deficiency), *Lancet* 1:239–241.

Gill, F. M., 1984, The natural history of factor VIII inhibitors in patients with hemophilia A, in: *Factor VIII Inhibitors* (L. W. Hoyer, ed.), pp. 19–29, Alan R. Liss, New York.

Ginsburg, D., Handin, R. I., Bonthron, D. T., Donlon, T. A., Bruns, G. A., Latt, S. A., and Orkin, S. H., 1985, Human Von Willebrand factor (VWF): Isolation of cDNA clones and chromosomal localization, *Science* 228:1401–1406.

Gitschier, J., Wood, W. I., Goralka, T. M., Wion, K. L., Chen, E. Y., Eaton, D. H., Vehar, G. A., Capon, D. J., and Lawn, R. M., 1984, Characterization of the human factor VIII gene, *Nature* 312:326–330.

Gitschier, J., Drayna, D., Tuddenham, E. G. D., White, R. I., and Lawn, R. M., 1985a, Genetic mapping and diagnosis of haemophilia A achieved through a *Bcl* I polymorphism in the factor VIII gene, *Nature* 314:738–740.

Gitschier, J., Lawn, R. M., Rotblat, F., Goldman, E., and Tuddenham, E. G. D., 1985b, Antenatal diagnosis and carrier detection of hemophilia A using factor VIII gene probe, *Lancet* 1:1093–1094.

Gitschier, J., Wood, W. I., Tuddenham, E. G. D., Shuman, M. A., Goralka, T. M., Chen, E. Y., and Lawn, R. M., 1985c, Detection and sequence of mutations in the factor VIII gene of haemophiliacs, *Nature* 315:427–430.

Gitschier, J., Wood, W. I., Shuman, M. A., and Lawn, R. M., 1986, Identification of a missense mutation in the factor VIII gene of a mild hemophiliac, *Science* 232:1415–1416.

Goodfellow, P. N., Davies, K. E., and Ropers, H. H., 1985, Report of the committee on the genetic constitution of the X and Y chromosomes, *Cytogenet. Cell. Genet.* 40:296–352.

Grunebaum, L., Cazenave, J. P., Camerino, G., Kloepfer, C., Mandel, J. L., Tolstoshev, P., Jaye, M., De la Salle, H., and Lecocq, J. P., 1984, Carrier detection of hemophilia B by using a restriction site polymorphism associated with the coagulation Factor IX gene, *J. Clin. Invest.* 73:1491–1495.

Harper, K., Winter, R. M., Pembrey, M. E., Hartley, D., Davies, K. E., and Tuddenham, E. G. D., 1984, A clinically useful DNA probe closely linked to hemophilia A, *Lancet* 2:6–8.

Hasan, H. J., Leonardi, A., Guerriero, G., Chelucci, C., Cianetti, L., Ciavarella, N., Ranieri, P., Pilolli, D., and Peschle, C., 1985, Hemophilia B with inhibitor: Molecular analysis of the subtotal deletion of the factor VIII gene, *Blood* 66:728–730.

Hay, C. W., Yong, S. L., Robertson, K. A., Linder, L., Growe, G. H., and McCillvray, R. T. A., 1986, Use of *Bam* HI polymorphism in the molecular analysis of hemophilia B in British Columbia, *Research* 16:183 (Abstract).

Hoyer, L. W., 1981, The factor VIII complex: Structure and function, *Blood* 58:1–13.

Jackson, C. M., and Nemerson, Y., 1980, Blood coagulation, *Annu. Rev. Biochem.* 49:765–811.

Janco, R. L., Phillips, J. A., Orlando, P., Davies, K. E., Old, J., and Antonarakis, S. E., 1986, Carrier testing strategy in hemophilia A, *Lancet* 1:148–149.

Jaye, M., de la Salle, H., Schamber, F., Balland, A., Kohli, V., Findeli, A., Tolstoshev, P., and Lecocq, J.-P., 1983, Isolation of a human anti-haemophilic factor

IX cDNA clone using a unique 52-base synthetic oligonucleotide probe deduced from the amino acid sequence of bovine factor XI, *Nucleic Acids Res.* 11:2325–2335.

Katayama, K., Ericsson, L. H., Enfield, D. L., Walsh, K. A., Neurath, H., Davie, E. W., and Titani, K., 1979, Comparison of amino acid sequence of bovine coagulation factor IX (Christmas factor) with that of other vitamin K-dependent plasma proteins, *Proc. Natl. Acad. Sci. USA* 76:4990–4994.

Keats, B., 1983, Genetic mapping: X chromosome, *Hum. Genet.* 64:28–32.

Kurachi, K., and Davie, E. W., 1982, Isolation and characterization of a cDNA coding for human factor IX, *Proc. Natl. Acad. Sci. USA* 79:6461–6464.

Lazarchick, J., and Hoyer, L. W., 1978, Immunoradiometric measurement of the factor VIII procoagulant antigen, *J. Clin. Invest.* 62:1048–1052.

Mattei, M. G., Baeteman, M. A., Heilig, R., Oberle, I., Davies, K., Mandel, J. L., and Mattei, J. F., 1985, Localization by *in situ* hybridization and the coagulation factor IX gene and of two polymorphic DNA probes with respect to the fragile X site, *Hum. Genet.* 69:327–331.

McKee, P. A., 1983, Haemostasis and disorders of blood coagulation, in: *The Metabolic Basis of Inherited Disease,* 5th ed. (J. B. Stanbury, J. B. Wyngaarden, D. S. Fredrickson, J. L. Goldstein, and M. S. Brown, eds.), pp. 1531–1560, McGraw-Hill, New York.

McKusick, V. A., 1962, On the X chromosome of man, *Q. Rev. Biol.* 37:69–175.

Noyes, C. M., Griffith, M. J., Roberts, H. R., and Lundblad, R. L., 1983, Identification of the molecular defect in factor IX Chapel Hill: Substitution of histidine for arginine at position 145, *Proc. Natl. Acad. Sci. USA* 80:4200–4202.

Oberle, I., Camerino, G., Heilig, R., Grunebaum, L., Cazenave, J. P., Crapanzano, C., Mannucci, P., and Mandel, J. L., 1985a, Genetic screening for hemophilia A with a polymorphic DNA probe, *N. Engl. J. Med.* 312:682–686.

Oberle, I., Drayna, D., Camerino, G., White, R., and Mandel, J. L., 1985b, The telomeric region of the human X chromosome long arm: Presence of a highly polymorphic DNA marker and analysis of recombination frequency, *Proc. Natl. Acad. Sci. USA* 82:2824–2828.

Oberle, I., Heilig, R., Moisan, J. P., Kloepfer, C., Mattei, M. G., Mattei, J. F., Bone, J., Froster-Iskenius, U., Jacobs, P. A., Lathrop, G. M., LaLouel, J. M., and Mandel, J. L., 1986, Genetic analysis of the fragile X mental retardation syndrome with two flanking polymorphic DNA markers, *Proc. Natl. Acad. Sci. USA* 83:1016–1020.

Peake, I. R., and Matthews, R. J., 1986, The prevalence of gene deletions in hemophilia B patients with inhibitors, *Ric. Clin. Lab.* 16:229 (Abstract).

Peake, I. R., Furlong, B. L., and Bloom, A. L., 1984, Carrier detection by gene analysis in a family with haemophilia B (factor IX deficiency), *Lancet* 1:242.

Phillips, D. G., Kazazian, H. H., Jr., Scott, A. F., Toole, J. J., and Antonarakis, S. E., 1985, Hemophilia A: Experience with prenatal diagnosis using DNA analysis, *Am. J. Hum. Genet.* 37:A224 (Abstract).

Purrello, M., Athadeff, B., Esposito, D., Szabo, P., Rocchi, M., Truett, M., Marsiarz, F., and Siniscalco, M., 1985, The human genes for hemophilia A and B flank the X chromosome fragile site at Xq27.3, *EMBO J.* 4:725–729.

Ratnoff, O. D., 1960, *Bleeding Syndromes: A Clinical Manual,* C. C. Thomas, Springfield, Illinois.

Rees, D. J. G., Rizza, C. R., and Brownlee, G. G., 1985, Haemophilia B caused by a point mutation in a donor splice junction of the human factor IX gene, *Nature* **316**:643–645.

Rotblat, F., O'Brien, D. P., O'Brien, F. J., Goodall, A. H., and Tuddenham, E. G., 1985, Purification of human factor VIII:C and its characterization by western blotting using monoclonal antibodies, *Biochemistry* **24**:4294–4300.

Toole, J. J., Knopf, J. L., Wozney, J. M., Sultzman, L. A., Buecher, J. L., Pittman, D. D., Kaufman, R. J., Brown, E., Shoemaker, C., Orr, E. C., Amphlett, G. W., Foster, W. B., Coe, M. L., Knudson, G. J., Fass, D. N., and Hewick, R. M., 1984, Molecular cloning of a cDNA encoding human anti-haemophilic factor, *Nature* **312**:342–347.

Vehar, G. A., Keyt, B., Eaton, D., Rodriguez, H., O'Brian, D. P., Rotblat, F., Oppermann, H., Keck, R., Wood, W. I., Harkins, R. N., Tuddenham, E. G. D., Lawn, R. M., and Capon, D. J., 1984, Structure of human factor VIII, *Nature* **312**:337–342.

Winship, P. R., Anson, D. S., Rizza, C. R., and Brownlee, G. G., 1984, Carrier detection in haemophilia B using two further intragenic restriction fragment length polymorphisms, *Nucleic Acids Res.* **12**:8861–8872.

Wion, K. L., Tuddenham, E. G. D., and Lawn, R. M., 1986, A new polymorphism in the factor VIII gene for prenatal diagnosis of hemophilia A, *Nucleic Acids, Res.* **14**:4535–4542.

Wood, W. I., Capon, D. J., Simonsen, C. C., Eaton, D. L., Gitschier, J., Keyt, B., Seeburg, P. H., Smith, D. H., Hollingshead, P., Wion, K. L., Delwart, E., Tuddenham, E. G. D., Vehar, G. A., and Lawn, R. M., 1984, Expression of active human factor VIII from recombinant DNA clones, *Nature* **312**:330–337.

Yoshitake, S., Schach, B. G., Foster, D. C., Davie, E. W., and Kurachi, K., 1985, Nucleotide sequence of the gene for human factor IX, *Biochemistry* **24**:3736–3750.

Youssoufian, H., Kazazian, H. H., Jr., Phillips, D. G., Aronis, S., Tsiftis, G., Brown, V. A., and Antonarakis, S. E., 1986, Recurrent mutations in hemophilia A: Evidence for CpG dinucleotides as mutation hotspots, *Nature* **324**:380–382.

Youssoufian, H., Antonarakis, S. E., Phillips, D. G., Aronis, S., Tsiftis, G., and Kazazian, H. H., Jr., 1987, Characterization of five partial deletions of the factor VIII gene:C gene, *Proc. Natl. Acad. Sci. USA* **84**:3772–3776.

Youssoufian, H., Antonarakis, S. E., Bell, W., Griffin, A. M., and Kazazian, H. H., 1988, Nonsense and missense mutations in hemophilia A: Estimate of the relative mutation rate at CG dinucleotides, *Am. J. Hum. Genet.* (in press).

Chapter 3

Cloning of the Duchenne/Becker Muscular Dystrophy Locus

Anthony P. Monaco

Division of Genetics and Mental Retardation Center
Children's Hospital
Department of Pediatrics
Harvard Medical School
Boston, Massachusetts 02115
and Program in Neuroscience
Harvard University
Cambridge, Massachusetts 02138

Louis M. Kunkel

Division of Genetics and Mental Retardation Center
Children's Hospital
Department of Pediatrics
Harvard Medical School
and Howard Hughes Medical Institute
Boston, Massachusetts 02115
and Program in Neuroscience
Harvard University
Cambridge, Massachusetts 02138

INTRODUCTION

The identification and molecular cloning of the Duchenne muscular dystrophy (DMD) gene represents the first step in the long path toward a basic understanding and potential therapy of this human genetic disorder. One of the most interesting challenges to modern medicine is to understand and alter the course of the many genetic disorders. There are more than 3000 known genetic disease phenotypes, yet the vast majority are poorly understood at the level of the underlying biochemical disturbance. The techniques of molecular biology have changed the way these disorders are analyzed, and presumably the next decade will see an explosion of new understanding in the various ways that genotype affects phenotype. Duchenne muscular dystrophy thus serves as an example of the prospects to come, and this review can serve as a guide toward similar work with other genetic disorders.

Background Information: Clinical Aspects of DMD

Duchenne muscular dystrophy (DMD) is a progressive muscle-wasting disorder inherited as an X-linked recessive trait. In all populations tested, approximately 1 of 3000 males is affected and one-third of cases are considered new or sporadic mutations (Moser, 1984). Penetrance in affected males is complete and female carriers are usually asymptomatic. Onset of DMD occurs before the age of 3 years with weakness of muscles surrounding the pelvic girdle. The muscle weakness results in difficulty in the child's ability to run and to get up from the floor. The proximal muscles are affected before the distal, with the lower limbs before the upper. There is fatty infiltration of the calves, giving rise to clinically detectable pseudohypertrophy. Muscle weakness is progressive, and loss of walking ability occurs by early adolescence, with confinement to a wheelchair for mobility. Eventually, the cardiac and truncal respiratory muscles are weakened, with death often resulting from respiratory infection and failure by the third decade. Mental retardation (I.Q. < 75) occurs in about 30% of DMD males, but does not seem to be progressive nor bear any correlation to the state or extent of the muscle weakness (Appel and Roses, 1983; Moser, 1984).

Becker muscular dystrophy (BMD) is a rarer muscle-wasting disorder inherited as an X-linked recessive trait, with the age of onset between 5 and 10 years. BMD patients exhibit clinical findings similar to those found in DMD, yet the overall course of the disease is less severe. Clinical studies have characterized a third set of patients, designated "outliers," with a clinical course intermediate in severity between DMD and BMD (Brooke *et al.*, 1983). Clinical heterogeneity has been suggested in a study of mentally handicapped DMD patients (Emery *et al.*, 1979). Mentally handicapped DMD patients seemed to have a milder clinical course than DMD patients of normal intelligence. Severely retarded patients rarely occurred in families with affected DMD males of normal intelligence.

Laboratory findings in both DMD and BMD males show increased serum activity (10- to 1000-fold) for the enzymes creatine-phosphokinase (CPK) and aldolase (Appel and Roses, 1983; Moser, 1984). In 70–80% of female carriers, moderate increases in serum enzyme activities can be detected. Muscle biopsy from DMD males is histologically characterized by progressive degeneration and random loss of muscle fibers with variation in fiber size (Dubowitz, 1985). Fiber type differentiation is impaired, and there is infiltration of fat and connective tissue. Most often, electromyogram and nerve conduction studies are undertaken to rule out Kugelberg–Welander disease (a progressive spinal muscle atrophy) and Pompe disease (a lysosomal acid maltase deficiency).

Background Information: Biochemical Aspects of DMD

Theories concerning the functional consequences of the primary genetic defect in DMD have centered around the "membrane theory" as an organizing pathophysiologic defect. The membrane theory states that the DMD gene defect decreases, abolishes, or makes abnormal an enzyme or structural protein that disrupts normal function of the muscle cell membrane to produce the symptomatic weakness and progressive degeneration (Rowland, 1980). This theory is attractive because it may account for the leakage of enzymes from muscle into blood serum detectable shortly after birth in affected males. This could occur in two ways that are not mutually exclusive: (1) physical holes in the membrane, and (2) altered permeability of the membrane. Physical holes in muscle membranes from DMD biopsy have been seen in electron microscopy studies and were called "delta lesions" (Mokri and Engel, 1975; Carpenter and Karpati, 1979). They occurred in both prenecrotic and necrotic muscle fibers and were shown to be permeable to horseradish peroxidase and procion yellow. Other electron microscopic studies of Duchenne muscle biopsy could not substantiate the sarcolemmal defects (Cullen and Fulthorpe, 1975). They did find, however, abnormal appearance of the sarcoplasmic reticulum, mitochrondria, and Z-lines of the sarcomere very early in the disease as well as regions of the fiber that were hypercontracted or overstretched.

Calcium homeostasis has been implicated for a possible role in the occurrence of opaque or hypercontracted fibers seen in DMD muscle biopsy (Cullen and Fulthorpe, 1975). A local increase of calcium influx without the proper intracellular buffering capacity could produce excessive contractions. These excessive contractions would stretch adjacent myofibrils, disrupt them, and initiate necrosis. Regeneration would be attempted, but could not keep up with the fairly constant rate of muscle fiber degeneration. Increased intracellular calcium could also activate proteases that would initiate necrosis and degeneration. One consistent finding in DMD muscle biopsy that lends support to the calcium theory is a problem with calcium regulation by the sarcoplasmic reticulum. Wood *et al.* (1978) used chemically skinned muscle fibers from Duchenne and normal muscle and found many Duchenne fibers that had a decrease in their ability to develop isometric tension. This could not be attributed to altered calcium levels nor altered substrate sensitivity of the contractile proteins, both of which were normal. Electron micrographs revealed disorientation of the myofiber structure that was hypothesized to contribute to the poor force development.

A reproducible defect in calcium metabolism has been shown in DMD cultured fibroblasts. The growth of DMD fibroblasts in calcium-deficient media was not inhibited as was the growth of normal fibroblasts (Fingerman *et al.*, 1984). This phenotypic cell-culture growth assay was used to distinguish accurately DMD versus control fibroblasts in ten samples tested blindly. The relevance of this phenotypic variation to the genotypic defect in DMD remains unclear. It must first be demonstrated that the calcium phenomenon is not a general characteristic of fibroblasts growing in the environment of Duchenne muscle degeneration and regeneration. In fact, an additional phenotypic difference in growth pattern of myoblasts cultured from Duchenne or normal males was attributed to the Duchenne-muscle environment and not to the primary genetic defect (Blau *et al.*, 1983; Webster *et al.*, 1986).

Problems with the study of membranes and intracellular calcium homeostasis in human muscle biopsy have made the elucidation of a specific biochemical defect in DMD very difficult. Contamination by fat and connective tissue membranes and differences in isolation and assay procedures between laboratories have made the search inconsistent. Many investigators turned to the erythrocyte membrane for a homogeneous population of membranes to study in DMD patients. Of 27 reported abnormalities in red blood cell membrane properties, all but one of 18 separate functions studied is not in question (Rowland, 1980).

Chromosomal Map Position

Because of the problems and inconsistencies encountered in the search for the DMD gene defect from a biochemical approach, attention turned to a search for the X-linked genetic locus encoding the DMD protein. The first evidence to sublocalize the DMD locus to a portion of the human X came from rare female cases that manifested the symptoms of DMD or BMD. Investigation of the chromosomes of these rare females indicated that each was a carrier of a balanced X;autosome translocation. In each case, the translocation breakpoint occurred in band Xp21 with no apparent preference for the autosomal breakpoint [for review see Boyd and Buckle (1986)]. A schematic example of one such case is given in Fig. 1. Here, using the X;21 translocation first described by Verellen-Dumoulin *et al.* (1984), the normal X chromosome was found to be late-replicating and therefore presumed to be the inactive X. The translocation chromosome was found to replicate early and was presumed to be the active X. It was assumed that with the normal X inactive and the Xp21 region of the X disrupted by the translocation, the DMD locus was unable to function properly and resulted in the phenotype of DMD. A similar inactivation pattern was observed in the other translocation females (Jacobs *et al.*, 1981), such that the

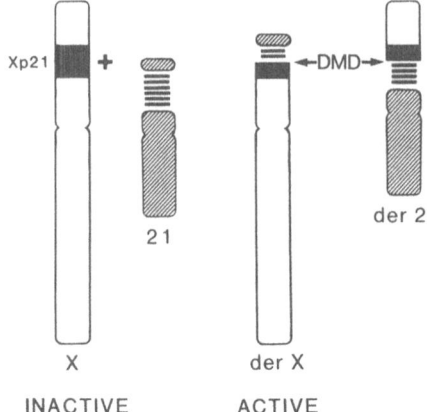

Fig. 1. Schematic representation of an X;autosome translocation in a BMD female. The ideograms of the X;21 balanced translocation in a female with BMD are demonstrated (Verellen-Dumoulin *et al.*, 1984). The translocation chromosome (derX) was found to be early-replicating and was assumed to be the active X chromosome, and the normal X was late-replicating.

combined evidence was that the Xp21 region must play a role in the etiology of the DMD and BMD phenotype.

Additional structural abnormalities that pinpointed Xp21 as the region of DMD included a number of cytologically visible deletions of the region. These were detected in male patients manifesting DMD associated with other X-linked disorders, such as adrenal hypoplasia (AH), glycerol kinase deficiency (GK), chronic granulomatous disease (CGD), retinitis pigmentosa (RP), and McLeod erythrocyte phenotype (McLeod) (Francke *et al.*, 1985; Baehner *et al.*, 1986; Bartley *et al.*, 1986). The first of these rare males described was the patient B.B., who exhibited DMD, CGD, and the McLeod red cell phenotype and a small interstitial deletion of Xp21 (Francke *et al.*, 1985). DNA isolated from a cell line established from the patient's lymphocytes could be demonstrated to indeed have a deletion, for the cloned DNA segment 754 (Hofker *et al.*, 1985) was found to be absent from this DNA sample. The remaining deletion patients were subsequently demonstrated to have DNA deletions of various other cloned segments, including sometimes the cloned probe 754.

The techniques of molecular biology opened the door to a more detailed molecular analysis of the Xp21 region. The demonstration that cloned segments of DNA were capable of detecting DNA sequence variation between individuals was one of these important developments (Kan and Dosy, 1978). It was proposed that these restriction fragment length polymorphisms (RFLP) (Botstein *et al.*, 1980) might enable the construction of a complete human linkage map. Most of the studies relevant to DMD made use of random DNA fragments isolated from flow-sorted human X-chromosome libraries (Davies *et al.*, 1981; Kunkel *et al.*, 1982; Hofker *et al.*, 1985). Many of these X-chromosome cloned DNA fragments were shown to detect RFLP alleles useful for genetic linkage analysis. In addition, most were physically mapped relative to various cytologically detected disruptions of X chromosomes which had been placed on rodent cell backgrounds. Segregation analysis of the random DNA loci defined by RFLP alleles in DMD families combined with physical mapping data consistently showed that the Xp21 region is the site for mutations causing both DMD and BMD (Davies *et al.*, 1983; Aldridge *et al.*, 1984; Kingston *et al.*, 1984; deMartinville *et al.*, 1985; Brown *et al.*, 1985; Dorkins *et al.*, 1985; Fadda *et al.*, 1985; Goodfellow *et al.*, 1985). The results of these studies are schematically outlined in Fig. 2. Here, the cloned probe physically closest to Xp21 is also genetically closest, and those flanking the Xp21 translocation breakpoints also could be shown to flank DMD and BMD mutations segregating in families.

STRATEGIES TO APPROACH THE GENE

Localization of the DMD/BMD locus to band Xp21 directed the search toward isolating and cloning sequences that mapped within this region. It was hoped that one cloned DNA fragment might be close enough to detect mutations in the DNA of patients. The general approach of isolating phage clones from flow-sorted human X-chromosome libraries to obtain DNA probes tightly linked to DMD had yielded the proximal clone 754 and several more distal probes, C7 [DXS28 (Dorkins *et al.*, 1985)] and B24 [DXS67 (Aldridge *et al.*, 1984)]. None of these randomly isolated DNA fragments was ge-

Anthony P. Monaco and Louis M. Kunkel

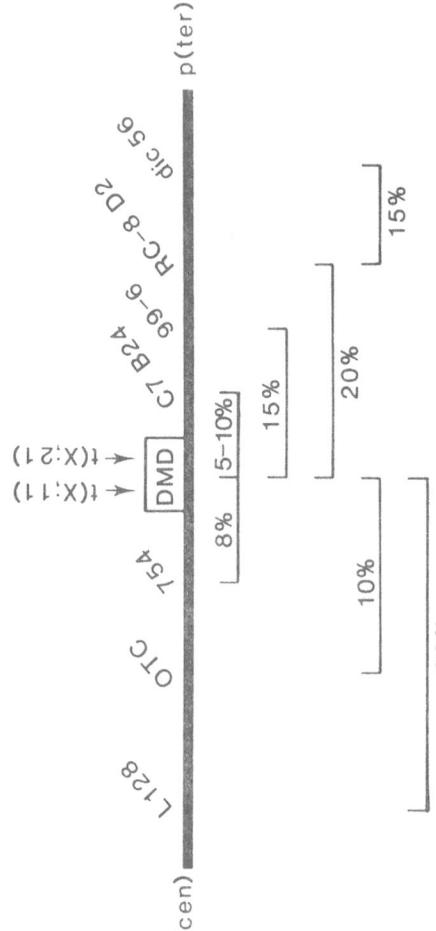

Fig. 2. Linkage relationships of Xp cloned loci and DMD mutations. The schematic map presents the relative physical order of several cloned loci from Xp21. A numerical estimate of their recombination distances to DMD mutations segregating in families at risk for DMD is given below. Two translocation breakpoints are indicated above the presumed location of the DMD locus.

netically or physically close enough to the DMD/BMD locus to study the mutant gene directly. In principle, additional clones could be obtained that might be closer, but alternative approaches were used to increase the chances of finding a close marker to DMD.

One quite straightforward strategy was to isolate the junction fragment from a translocation chromosome in a female with muscular dystrophy. If the breakpoint on the autosome involved DNA already isolated, then this cloned DNA might allow the detection and cloning of the breakpoint. The translocation demonstrated in Fig. 1 was a candidate for this approach. In this patient the autosomal breakpoint was in the 28S ribosomal locus on chromsome 21 (Verellen-Dumoulin *et al.*, 1984). A ribosomal DNA probe from this region on chromosome 21 revealed an altered-size *Bam*HI fragment on Southern blot analysis of DNA from the affected female (Worton *et al.*, 1984). This altered-size *Bam*HI fragment was presumed to contain DNA from both chromosome 21 and Xp21 connected by the translocation event. The *Bam*HI junction fragment was recovered from a genomic phage library constructed from a somatic cell hybrid bearing the human X;21 translocation chromosome on a rodent chromosome background (Ray *et al.*, 1985). By comparing the restriction pattern of the junction fragment to normal DNA on chromosome 21, the exact breakpoint was determined and an Xp21-specific DNA fragment was isolated from the other side. Since the translocation break seemed to cause DMD, potentially the X-chromosome portion of the cloned junction might reside within the DMD gene.

A second strategy involved a different visible chromosome abnormality, an interstitial deletion of the Xp21 region in a male patient, B.B., who exhibited four X-linked disorders: DMD, CGD, RP, and the McLeod red blood cell phenotype (Francke *et al.*, 1985). The DNA isolated from B.B. was tested by hybridization for more than 30 cloned fragments from Xp, some of which are indicated on Fig. 2. The only clone shown to be absent from B.B.'s DNA was the Xp21 locus DXS84, defined by the random probe 754 (Francke *et al.*, 1985; Hofker *et al.*, 1985). The probe 754 exhibits 5–10% recombination with DMD mutations segregating in families and was used along with other Xp probes that detect RFLPs in preliminary studies of carrier detection and prenatal diagnosis (Bakker *et al.*, 1985).

The approach taken by Kunkel *et al.* (1985*b*) was to saturate the Xp21 region specifically with cloned DNA fragments using DNA isolated from B.B. as a guide. DNA isolated from a lymphoblastoid cell line from the patient B.B. was used in a competitive reassociation and cloning strategy to yield a recombinant plasmid library highly enriched for DNA segments missing from the Xp21 deletion in this patient (Kunkel *et al.*, 1985*b*). A 200:1 excess of sheared DNA from B.B. was denatured and then reassociated under accelerated conditions [phenol emulsion reassociation technique, pERT (Kohne *et al.*, 1977)] with a trace amount of *Mbo*I-cleaved DNA isolated from a 49,XXXXY human lymphoblastoid cell line. The pERT conditions allowed the reaction to reach Cot values (Britten and Kohne, 1968; Wetmur and Davidson, 1968) necessary for unique sequence fragments present in the trace *Mbo*I-cleaved DNA to reassociate. The general cloning strategy using molecules with different types of termini had been previously described for isolating moderately repeated segments from the mouse Y chromosome (Lamar and Palmer, 1984). It allows only those fragments from the *Mbo*I-cleaved tracer DNA that escaped reassociation with complementary sequences in the sheared driver DNA to reassociate with their correct complementary strand of *Mbo*I-cleaved DNA. These latter double-stranded molecules have *Mbo*I ends compatible with ligation in the *Bam*HI site of the plasmid vector pBR322 (Bolivar *et al.*, 1977). The vast majority of other reassociated molecules do not have intact *Mbo*I ends because one or both of the complementary strands are from the sheared driver DNA. Analysis of over 400 plasmid clones from this pERT library has yielded nine DNA fragments absent from the DNA of B.B., the patient from whose DNA the library was constructed.

The large Xp21 deletion in the DNA of the patient B.B. was estimated to encompass two to ten million base pairs (Francke *et al.*, 1985). Contained within this region were several structural breakpoints segregated in rodent–human somatic cell hybrids that helped subdivide the pERT clones and the probe 754. The nine absent pERT clones as well as previously described random clones are schematically presented in Fig. 3 and mapped relative to various breakpoints within the region. Five clones (pERT55, pERT145, pERT378, pERT379, and pERT634) were present in the DNA from a rodent–human cell hybrid that contained a human X chromosome presumed to be intact from Xp11.3 to Xqter, but which may actually have broken closer to Xp21 (Wieacker *et al.*, 1984). Therefore, these five DNA probes all mapped proximal (toward the centromere) from this breakpoint. Three clones [pERT469, 754 (DXS84), and pERT84] were absent from the DNA in the Xp11.3 hybrid, yet were present in the DNA from two somatic cell hybrids that contained a human X chromosome intact from Xp21 to Xqter. The two Xp21 translocation breakpoints, one to chromosome 21 (Verellen-Dumoulin, 1984) and the other to chromosome 11 (Greenstein *et al.*, 1980), gave rise to the phenotype of DMD in females bearing the translocations. Only one probe (pERT87) was absent from the DNA in hybrids, each containing one of these translocation chromosomes, but was present as two-copy hybridization in DNA isolated from a fibroblast cell line (Fryns *et al.*, 1982) that contained a heterozygous deletion from Xp21 to Xpter. This result mapped pERT87 distal (toward the telomere) to the X;21 and X;11 translocation breakpoints, yet proximal to both the B.B. deletion and the terminal deletion breakpoints. More recently the relative order of the various clones (centromere to telomere) has been independently confirmed from studies of patients with large Xp21 deletions and DMD associated with glycerol kinase deficiency, adrenal hypoplasia (van Ommen *et al.*, 1986; Bertelson *et al.*, 1986; Francke *et al.*, 1987), McLeod phenotype, and CGD (Bertelson *et al.*, 1987). The mapping of cloned probes and disease loci is given in Fig. 3.

DETECTION OF DELETIONS IN DMD AND BMD PATIENTS

One of the ways by which mutant phenotypes can be generated is deletion of the genomic locus encoding a particular product. In two X-linked disorders, Lesch–Nyhan syndrome (Yang *et al.*, 1984)

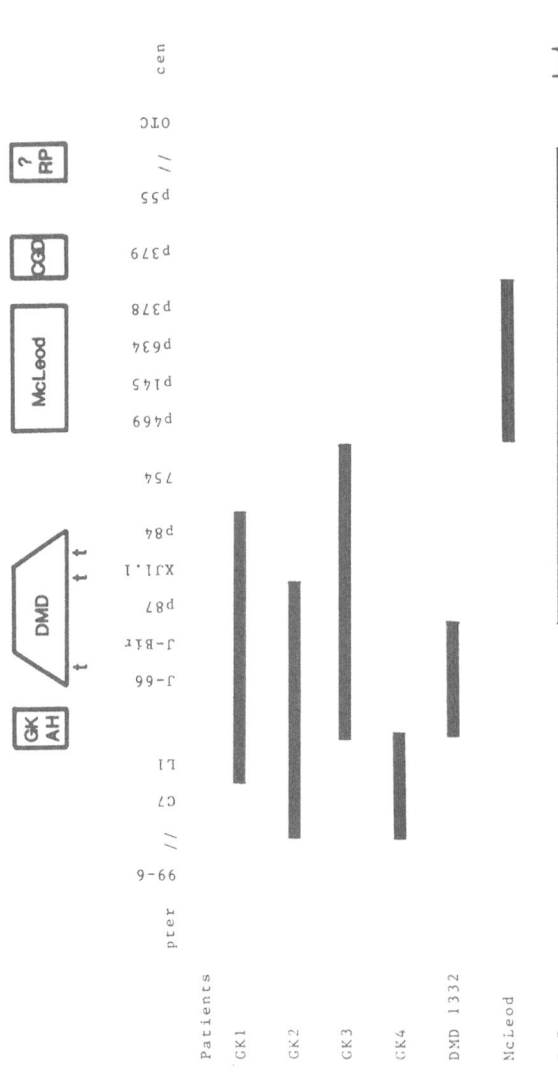

Fig. 3. Schematic map of Xp21 disease loci and cloned loci. The relative positions of various Xp21-cloned segments are given (central section of the figure) and were established by hybridizing cloned segments to DNA samples isolated from patients with deletions and translocations associated with various X-linked disorders (Bertelson *et al.*, 1986, 1987; Francke *et al.*, 1987). Many positions were confirmed by hybridization of cloned segments to DNA samples isolated from rodent–human hybrid cell lines that had lost various sections of the X-chromosome short arm (Kunkel *et al.*, 1985*b*; Monaco and Kunkel, 1987; Monaco *et al.*, 1987). By the presence or absence of various cloned segments from these DNA samples, the minimum region of deletion overlap can be deduced and the relative order of the loci established. The genetic disease loci are depicted and the DNA clones that are deleted in each disorder and the extent of each deletion are depicted below. Scale bar: approximately 1 mb.

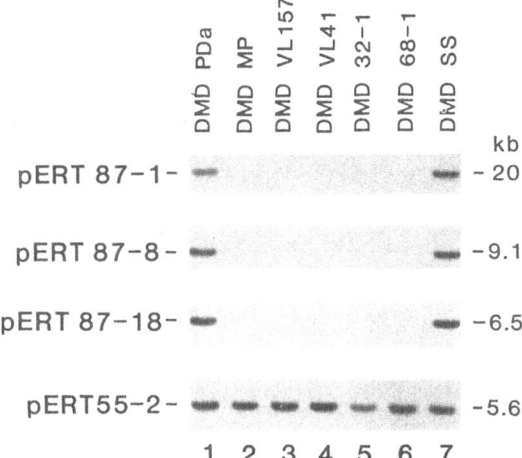

Fig. 4.   Southern blot analysis of DNA from seven males with DMD. Lanes 1–7 contain *Pst*I-digested DNA from the patients. Two identical nitrocellulose filters were hybridized with pERT87-18 and pERT87-1. The same filters were then rehybridized with pERT87-8 and pERT55-2, respectively. The autoradiographs are presented as separate segments of each original autoradiograph. The fragment hybridized is indicated to the left of the figure; the sizes of hybridizing fragments are indicated on the right and were calculated from ^{32}P-end-labeled, *Hind*III-cleaved lambda DNA. The designation above each lane is the nomenclature for each DMD male.

and ornithine transcarbamylase deficiency (OTC) (Rozen *et al.*, 1985), 18 and 6.6% of patients were found to have partial or complete deletions of genomic sequences complementary to the cloned cDNAs for hypoxanthine-guanine phosphoribosyltransferase and OTC, respectively. On a theoretical basis, eight DNA probes from a small region of the genome (defined by the B.B. deletion) should increase the probability that one probe will detect a deletion at a specific disease locus if such deletions exist (Lange *et al.*, 1985). Therefore, the original seven pERT clones and the probe 754 were used to search for microdeletions in the DNA isolated from DMD males. Initially, 57 unrelated DMD males were tested by hybridization with the eight Xp21 probes and only one probe, pERT87, was found to be deleted in five of these 57 males (Monaco *et al.*, 1985), and an example of these deletions is given in Fig. 4. Of 61 normal X chromosomes tested, no deletions were found with any of the eight Xp21 probes. The Xp21-specific DNA fragment isolated from the X;21 translocation junction (XJ) was also found to detect deletions in DMD males and was presumed to be in close proximity to pERT87 (Ray et al., 1985).

The structural alterations detected by the pERT87 probe indicated physical closeness to the DMD locus, but formal genetic linkage analysis was needed with cloned DNA fragments from within the deleted region. Therefore, extensive chromosome walking (Bender et al., 1983) was undertaken from the original 200 base pair pERT87 probe to determine the extent of the deletions and to obtain RFLP detecting probes. Chromosome walking was accomplished by hybridization (Benton and Davis, 1977) of the small pERT87 clone to a human partial digest recombinant phage library. Hybridizing phage were plaque purified and DNA prepared. The human DNA insert was cleaved with restriction endonucleases and the position of various sites established relative to each other (a map was created). All portions of the human insert DNA were subcloned in plasmid vectors and tested for hybridization on genomic Southern blots for an Xp21-specific pattern. The repeat versus unique sequence status of the subclones was also established in this manner. The subclones from each end of the first walk were used as hybridization probes back against the human recombinant library and newly hybridizing phage identified. Those that extended in one direction (had one probe present but not the other), were plaque purified and DNA isolated. Restriction enzyme maps of the new human inserts were compared to the previous map and the degree of overlap established. By successive cycles of library screening and restriction enzyme mapping, nine bidirectional walks were accomplished in partial digest phage libraries and eventually yielded clones distributed over a total of 220 kilobases (kb) of DNA (designated the DXS164 locus) (Goodfellow et al., 1985). The complete 220 kb (schematically demonstrated in Fig. 5) of genomic DNA around the pERT87 probe was subcloned into plasmid vectors, and all unique-sequence subclones tested by hybridization on Southern blots for Xp21 localization.

Single-copy clones from the DXS164 locus were used to search for RFLPs in DNA samples isolated from four females cleaved with 24 restriction enzymes [for RFLP search strategy, see Aldridge et

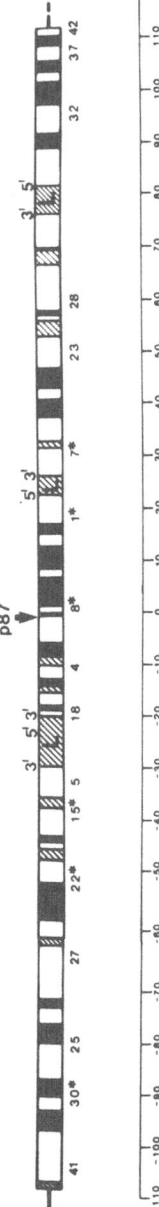

Fig. 5.   Schematic map of 220 kb of the DXS164 locus. The map of the DXS164 locus is subdivided into highly repeated regions indicated by dark boxes, moderately repeated regions (a unique Xp21 band among many other hybridizing fragments) by hatched boxes, single-copy subclones by white boxes, and the LINE sequence (Singer, 1982) by an L. The numerical designations of unique subclones are indicated below their corresponding map position and those that recognize RFLPs are marked with an asterisk. The LINE sequences were further characterized as to their length and directionality using cloned 5' and 3' ends of a human LINE sequence as hybridization probes (provided by B. Schmeckpeper) as indicated above the map. The centromere of the X chromosome is oriented toward the right of the figure and the terminus toward the left. A kilobase scale is given beneath the schematic.

al. (1984)]. From this search, seven different DNA clones were found that recognized a total of 13 RFLPs (indicated with asterisks in Fig. 5). Three of the DXS164 clones that detected the most informative RFLPs (pERT87-1, -8, and -15) were distributed for a large international study of DMD and BMD patients (Kunkel *et al.*, 1986). The DNA of 1346 DMD and BMD males was tested for deletions, and 88 (6.5%) were found to be deleted for one or more of the three DXS164 clones. No deletion has been detected in a normal male, indicating that the deletion represents the primary mutation event resulting in the disorder. The DNA from 55 patients identified as deletions in the large collaborative study was tested for the presence or absence of sequences from the 220 kb of the DXS164 locus (Monaco *et al.*, 1987). Twenty-five deletions had one breakpoint in cloned DNA, with overlapping and nonoverlapping deletions extending in both directions relative to the DXS164 restriction map. Most DMD deletions extended for more than 100 kb with neither breakpoint within cloned DNA, and only four deletions had both endpoints within the DXS164 locus. One of these four was a small deletion (about 6 kb) identified in a BMD patient (Hart *et al.*, 1987*a,b*). The other three deletions with both endpoints in the DXS164 locus were identified in DMD patients. The DMD and BMD deletions had overlapping regions of deficiency, and there were two large BMD deletions that extended off the DXS164 locus.

Clearly, the DNA clones derived from the DXS164 locus identified DNA sequences within or closely associated with the DMD locus, and a number of them are used for prenatal diagnosis and carrier detection of DMD mutations. Yet, recombinants are observed (5–6%) between DXS164-derived clones that detect RFLPs and DMD and BMD mutations segregating in families (Kunkel *et al.*, 1986; Fischbeck *et al.*, 1986). This evidence suggested that the DMD/BMD gene was very large or the region containing it was recombining at a very high rate.

The DXS164 locus appeared to be centrally located with regard to deletion events that give rise to DMD and BMD. From genetic linkage studies and observed recombinants between DXS164 and DMD mutations, the Xp21 locus involved in muscular dystrophy seemed to be extremely large or possibly outside the DXS164 locus.

Therefore, several deletion junction fragments were isolated to obtain DNA on the other side of the breakpoint an unknown distance away. Deletion breakpoints near unique-sequence clones of the DXS164 locus were identified on Southern blots as altered-size restriction fragments. Junction fragments from four of these breakpoints were recovered in genomic phage libraries constructed from deletion DNA samples. The individual deletion libraries were screened with the DXS164 clone that had recognized the altered-size junction fragment on the Southern blot. The breakpoints of four large deletions were isolated in this manner, and the new loci (depicted schematically relative to the DXS164 locus in Figs. 3 and 6) were physically mapped relative to the translocation breakpoints in Xp21 that had been segregated in rodent–human somatic cell hybrids (Monaco *et al.*, 1987). The DXS164 locus had previously been mapped on the distal side of both the X;21 and X;11 translocation breakpoints (Kunkel *et al.*, 1985*b*), yet two of the new outlying deletion breakpoint loci (J-MD and J-47) were demonstrated to map on the proximal side of the X;21 translocation breakpoint (toward the centromere), yet still distal to the X;11 breakpoint. The other two loci defined by deletion junction clones, J-Bir and J-66, have breakpoints in the DXS164 locus toward the opposite end of the locus from those of J-MD and J-47, and therefore extend toward the telomere of the short arm. The outlying junction fragments from the deletions were used for chromosomal walking in normal DNA and tested against other DMD deletions and translocation breakpoints (Monaco *et al.*, 1987). These outlying regions added to the number of cloned loci capable of detecting DMD mutations.

One of the more interesting features of the various deletions was the observation that some of the deletions were inherited in an unusual pattern. In some cases two offspring would inherit deletions from a mother who was not herself heterozygous for a deletion mutation. In some cases the deletion could be definitely traced to maternal gametic origin, one to paternal and the remainder were of undistinguishable origin (Bakker *et al.*, 1987; Darras and Francke, 1987). The most likely explanation is germ-line mosaicism, that is, a deletion produced in mitotic proliferation of primitive germ cells, which then can be inherited by more than one individual in the next

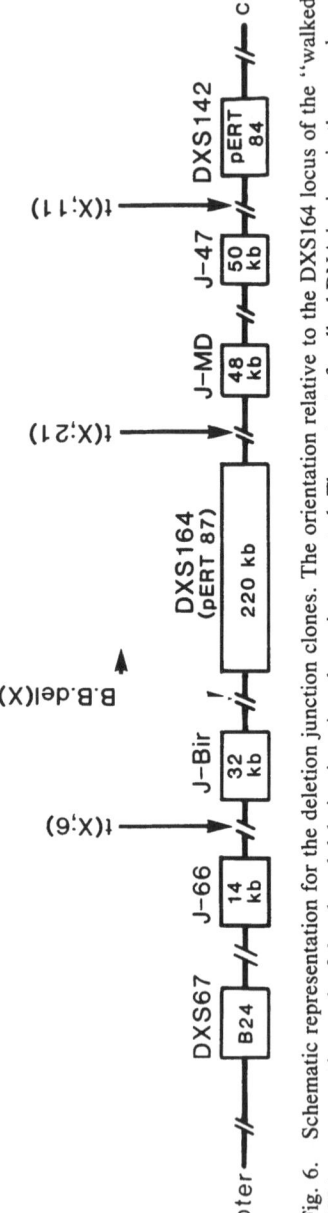

Fig. 6. Schematic representation for the deletion junction clones. The orientation relative to the DXS164 locus of the "walked" DNA encompassing each of the cloned deletion junction clones is presented. The extent of walked DNA is given in the open boxes. The B.B. deletion breakpoint is indicated, and three translocation breakpoints are also given (Monaco et al., 1987). Two other Xp21 loci, DXS67 and DXS142, are also indicated. The breaks in the lines indicate that DNA distances are unknown. The centromere of the X is indicated to the right and the terminus to the left.

generation. Consistent with the hypothesis was the identification of an identical deletion junction fragment in one such family. This would indicate that inherited deletions arose from the same event in the germ line of the mother. The unusual inheritance of maternal origin deletions and the fact that some deletions are clearly paternal in origin might indicate that the majority of deletions arise as mitotic events and not meiotic events. However, the fact of unusual inheritance must be considered in determining the risk of having another DMD male in a family with one affected male and no previous family history.

IDENTIFICATION OF THE DMD TRANSCRIPT

To identify DNA clones derived from the DXS164 locus that might contain exons of the DMD gene, a search was initiated for sequences conserved among different mammalian species. This strategy was conceived based on the evidence that DNA sequences encoding for amino acids (exons) have been conserved in the evolution of mammalian species, while noncoding sequences (introns) have diverged over time (Perler *et al.*, 1980). The search for conserved sequences yielded two DNA fragments, separated by more than 70 kb in the DXS164 restriction map, that hybridized at high stringency to DNA isolated from all mammalian species (Monaco *et al.*, 1986). The two mouse loci equivalent to the human conserved fragments were recovered from a mouse genomic phage library and the loci mapped to the mouse X chromosome. The nucleotide sequences of both the human and mouse conserved regions were determined, and each was found to contain the structure for an exon with short open reading frames bounded by potential 5′ splice, 3′ splice, and lariat consensus sequences (Monaco *et al.*, 1986). From the orientation of the potential 5′ and 3′ splice sites in the human genomic sequence and the relation of this sequence to the restriction map of the DXS164 locus, the direction of transcription across both open reading frames was predicted to be from the centromere to the telomere of the short arm.

The nucleotide sequence predicted that both conserved regions were potential exons which might be represented in an RNA transcript. Northern blots (Thomas, 1980) of RNA isolated from a variety of human cell lines and fetal tissue were prepared and hybridized with the two conserved potential exons. One of the human DNA fragments (pERT87-25) detected a large 16-kb transcript in both poly A + and total RNA samples isolated from human fetal skeletal muscle. A poly A + RNA sample in which the transcript could be detected served as a template in the construction of a cDNA library (Gubler and Hoffman, 1983; Huynh *et al.*, 1985; Monaco *et al.*, 1986). The library was screened with the exon containing genomic DNA fragments, and cDNA clones corresponding to approximately 10% of the large muscle-derived transcript were obtained. Hybridization of the cDNA clones to genomic DNA samples and the overlapping phage clones derived from the entire DXS164 locus indicated that the partial cDNA was encoded by a minimum of eight small exons spanning more than 130 kb of genomic DNA. The extensive spreading of the small exons predicted that the entire 16-kb transcript might be encoded from exons distributed over one to two million base pairs of genomic DNA.

Using the original partial human cDNA, it was possible to obtain the entire cDNA representation of the human transcript (Koenig *et al.*, 1987). The full length encompasses 14 kb of DNA, slightly less than the original estimate of 16 kb from Northern blot analysis. The human partial cDNA was also used to screen both mouse cardiac and skeletal muscle cDNA libraries, and approximately one-half of the mouse equivalent DMD transcript has also been obtained from these sources. Northern blots were prepared from multiple RNA samples isolated from different tissues and developmental stages in the mouse. The mouse expresses a similar 16-kb transcript in both adult and neonatal muscle tissues. The transcript is observed in both cardiac and skeletal muscle of mouse as well as on an RNA sample isolated from 15-day combined gravid uterus and placenta (Hoffman *et al.*, 1987). Additional experiments using human cardiac samples have also confirmed the presence of the DMD transcript in cardiac tissue. The expression of the DMD gene in cardiac tissue presumably explains the cardiac involvement in many patients with DMD. The inability to detect transcription in other tissues indicates that the

DMD transcript was below the level of detection and does not exclude the possibility that other tissues have very low levels of gene expression. Even in muscle RNA samples, the DMD transcript is approximately 1/500 of the expression of tubulin. The tissue distribution of the DMD gene is consistent with the manifestation of the disorder, and the means by which this gene results in disease will have to await further studies with the DMD protein.

THE DMD LOCUS

The total of cloned DNA sequences derived from the DXS164 locus and the three junction loci of J-Bir, J-MD, and J-47 is 350 kb. The XJ locus (DXS206) isolated from the X;21 translocation breakpoint (Ray et al., 1985) has been expanded by chromosome walking in genomic phage libraries to 160 kb. It was shown to overlap the centromere side of the DXS164 locus and the telomere side of the J-MD locus using cloned fragments from the extreme ends of these two loci (Burghes et al., 1987). The total of 510 kb is the minimum of cloned Xp21 DNA that is structurally altered in DMD and BMD males. These same DNA loci were used to create a long-range restriction map of the Xp21 region using pulsed-field gel electrophoresis (PFGE) (Schwartz and Cantor, 1984; Carle et al., 1986) and restriction enzymes that cut at rare sites in the genome. Several groups have completed a long-range restriction map of over 4000 kb of the Xp21 region using DNA probes derived from the DXS164 locus, J-66, J-Bir, J-MD, J-47, and XJ (DXS206). The results confirm that the DMD/BMD locus could potentially span 2000 kb (van Ommen et al., 1986; Burmeister and Lehrach, 1986; Kenwrick et al., 1987; van Ommen et al., 1987). The megabase map indicates that the X;6 and X;11 translocation breakpoints, known from cytological analysis and physical mapping (Boyd et al., 1987) to be separated by a large distance, are in fact more than 1000 kb apart.

From double digests with SfiI and several restriction enzymes whose target sites contain CpG dinucleotides, a clustering of CpG sites was mapped using PFGE near the loci detected by J-47 and pERT84 (Burmeister and Lehrach, 1986). Such clusters of CpG dinucleotides are characteristic of HTF islands (*Hpa*II tiny fragments) that have been found at the 5' end of many genes (Brown and Bird, 1986). The suggestion that the 5' end of the DMD gene is located in the vicinity of the HTF island is consistent with the direction of transcription established for the 16-kb muscle transcript.

The early results indicated that the DMD/BMD locus might be very large. With the entire cDNA available, an actual estimate can be made for the size of the genomic locus. The entire cDNA restriction enzyme map is given alongside a genomic locus map in Fig. 7. Subclones of the cDNA (given in numerical order on the left of the figure) were individually radiolabeled and hybridized either to phage DNA digests of walked DNA at various loci or to deletion DNA samples. More than 50 uniquely hybridizing *Hind*III fragments were demonstrated, and their approximate positions are given relative to the known points within Xp21. The most 5' exon of the gene was mapped within the walked DNA of the DXS142 (pERT84) locus, which had previously been mapped as centromeric relative to the X;11 translocation breakpoint. The fifth exon could be mapped to the walked DNA of the J-MD locus, with four exons falling between DXS142 and J-MD, but none were localized within the J-47 locus. The genomic distances between these loci are not known exactly, but minimum distances are indicated on the locus kilobase scale. A single *Hind*III fragment could be positioned within the walks of the

---

Fig. 7. Physical maps of the Duchenne muscular dystrophy cDNA and gene. (a) Human cDNA fragments used as probes in this study (enumerated according to their position along the cDNA map; i.e., sequences between the (*n*-1)th and *n*th kb define probe *n*). (b) the extent of 53 DMD deletions relative to the cDNA map; each line represents one deletion; dashed lines indicate uncertainty of the deletion breakpoint for deletions analyzed only with Xp21 genomic probes (analyzed prior to the cDNA cloning). (c) cDNA restriction map. (d) Brackets show portions of the cDNA detecting single *Hind*III genomic fragments (generally the limits of portions are only indicative). When known, the position of these *Hind*III fragments along the genomic map is indicated. The position of the third *Hind*III fragment (4.2 kb) distal to J-47 has been deduced from the analysis of a DMD deletion. Horizontal dashes indicate precise localization of coding sequences in cloned genomic sequences. (e) Genomic physical map: black bars, cloned genomic sequences; arrows, translocation or deletion breakpoints.

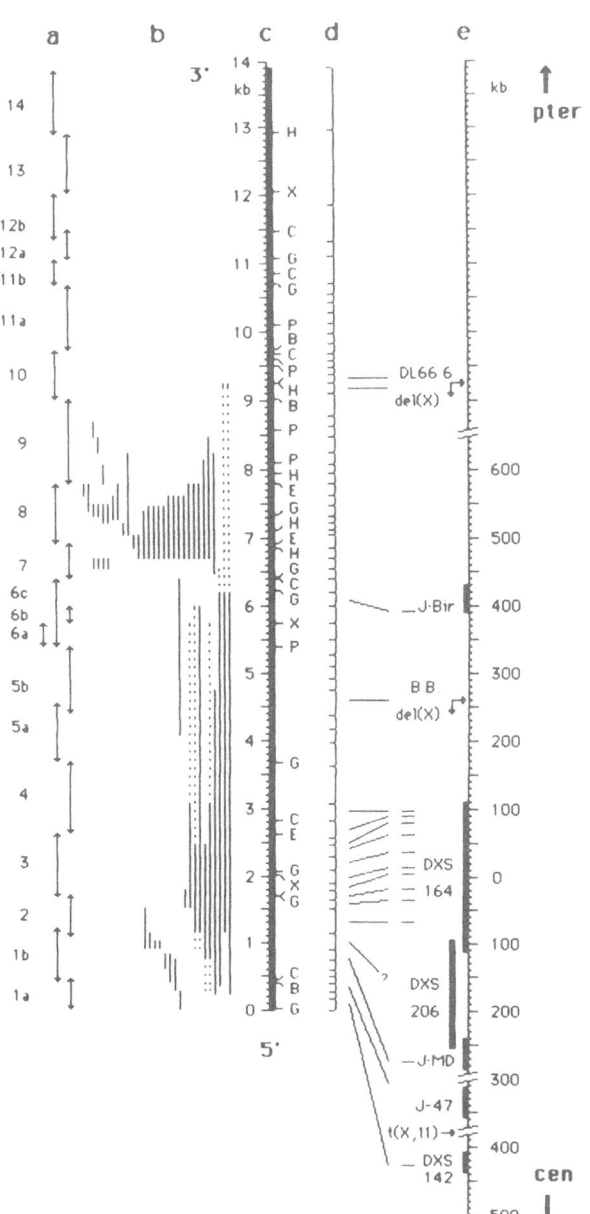

DXS206 locus [there are actually two exons within this *Hind*III fragment (Burghes *et al.*, 1987)]. Twelve exons have been mapped to the walks of the DXS164 (pERT87) locus, and these approximate positions are indicated on the figure. A minimum of five exons do not hybridize to the DXS164 locus, but are absent from the DNA of B.B. The next exon detects a junction fragment in the DNA of B.B., with four more *Hind*III fragments centromeric to the J-Bir locus. The 33rd hybridizing *Hind*III fragment can be positioned in the phage walks surrounding J-Bir. The J-Bir locus has been estimated by pulsed field gel electrophoresis to be approximately 300 kb from the last subclone of the DXS164 locus, with the B.B. deletion breakpoint falling halfway between them. From the combined information, the first 6.5 kb of the DMD cDNA is encoded by a minimum of 33 exons spaced over a minimum of 900 kb of human genomic DNA.

The remainder of the human cDNA is more difficult to map. The single reference point is the J-66 locus, which has been estimated to be 800 kb from the J-Bir locus (G.-J.B. van Ommen *et al.*, 1987). The last 4.5 kb of the human cDNA is not deleted from the DL66.6 DNA sample, yet the cDNA from 6.5 to 9.5 kb is deleted. This indicates that the exons encoding this 3 kb of cDNA span a distance of 800 kb. The remaining exons from 9.5 to 14 kb are probably spread over an equivalent distance, and this, combined with the other mapping information, indicates that the DMD locus is greater than two million base pairs of genomic DNA. The large size of the DMD locus is consistent with the high new mutation frequency of the locus, the heterogeneity of translocation breakpoints in female patients, and the extent and frequency of deletion mutations.

As described in an earlier section (pp. 72–73), deletions were detected in the DNA of patients using both the pERT87 subclones and the XJ1.1 clone. Both cloned regions (see Fig. 7) are located on the 5' end of the gene and thus potentially detect deletions only in this region of the locus. Using the entire cDNA as a hybridization probe, an analysis of patients not previously demonstrated to bear deletions has indicated that many more deletions can represent the primary mutation in DMD patients. Greater than 50% of all DMD patients bear deletions of DNA somewhere within the locus (Koenig *et al.*, 1987; Forrest *et al.*, 1987). In the families where deletions are detected, prediction for the inheritance of DMD is highly accurate. The remaining 50% of families must rely on RFLP detecting probes from within or surrounding the locus. The large size of the locus renders it subject to recombination events within the locus, which has led to problems in prediction for the inheritance of the DMD or BMD chromosome, especially when probes from only one side of the locus are used (Francke *et al.*, 1987). The full-length cDNA, which has exons spread over the entire gene, should soon yield the necessary RFLP alleles to mark both ends and the center of the gene. This should eliminate some of the problems from recombination across the locus, for at least these events can be accurately traced.

   One of the interesting questions relevant to the DMD locus is why deletions of various genomic exons yield phenotypes so different in severity (BMD and DMD can both be caused by deletions). One of the possible mechanisms concerns the structure of the exons lost in the deletion event. The DNA sequences surrounding all of the exons from within the DXS164 locus have been determined and compared to the sequence of the cDNA (Monaco *et al.*, 1988). Of the exons currently sequenced, they have been observed to begin and end at all three positions of triplet codons. This phenomenon has been well documented in the rat embryonic myosin genomic sequences (Strehler *et al.*, 1986). The observation that the DMD exons begin and end in all three positions of the triplet codon presented a possible molecular explanation for deletions of the DXS164 locus found in both DMD and BMD patients. The phenotypic differences might be due to the resulting pattern of exons brought together by the deletion event. A DMD deletion might connect two genomic regions that contain exons not compatible with the maintenance of an open reading frame in the resulting spliced mRNA. The nucleotide triplet code would be frameshifted, and an eventual stop codon would truncate the protein during translation. A BMD deletion might connect genomic exons that maintain the same triplet codon reading frame in the spliced mRNA. The mRNA would translate into a protein with an interstitial deletion of amino acid sequences, thus resulting in a semifunctional protein and a milder clinical phenotype.

Three DMD deletions that break around sequenced exons were found to connect genomic regions containing one exon that breaks between triplets and another exon that breaks within the triplet codon, thus shifting the mRNA open reading frame (Monaco et al., 1988). Three BMD deletions remove genomic exons which begin and end between triplet codons. The deletions connect two exons in the resulting mRNA that would maintain an open reading frame. For one small BMD deletion (#68), the number of deleted amino acids in the translated protein would be 40. The amino acid residues that are connected together in the small deletion maintain not only the open reading frame of the protein, but also the periodicity of the heptad repeat (a-b-c-d-e-f-g) found at the intron:exon border (see next section). Another BMD deletion was very large (>180 kb) and was also found to be missing the J-Bir locus. The deletion begins with an exon that breaks between a triplet codon and would have an observed probability of 66% that the unknown exon to which it connects is also breaking between triplets. This would create a larger interstitial deletion in the protein, which might cause a less severe clinical phenotype than a truncated protein at the same point. This BMD patient is also more severely affected clinically than the BMD patient with the small deletion (Hart et al., 1987a,b). To test this hypothesis, the genomic exon sequence for the other side of the deletion is currently being sequenced.

The pattern of genomic exon splice sites in the DXS164 locus also predicts that point mutations that prevent splicing would result in the deletion of different single exons or the inclusion of introns in the resulting mRNA. A large percentage of nondeletion mutations in the DMD/BMD locus might be splice site mutants [about 48% in the thalassemias (Orkin and Kazazian, 1984)]. The small size of the exons predicts that the ratio of nucleotides involved in splicing to the exon mutation target is larger than in most genes. The number of single exons in the DXS164 locus with one end breaking inside a triplet codon is 7 of 11. Therefore, the majority of splice site mutations would result in a truncated protein because of frameshift in the spliced mRNA. These might cause the more severe DMD phenotype, while splice mutations involving exons with both ends between triplet codons would result in the BMD phenotype.

One of the most perplexing questions is the cause of mental retardation seen in about one-third of muscular dystrophy patients (Moser, 1984). Originally, the 14-kb transcript was found in skeletal, cardiac, and smooth muscle tissues from humans and mice by Northern blot analysis of RNA (Monaco *et al.*, 1986; Hoffman *et al.*, 1987*a*). More recently, with the use of more sensitive ribonuclease protection assays, the DMD gene has been shown to be expressed in brain tissue of mice and rats as well as differentiated muscle cells in culture (Chamberlain *et al.*, 1988; Nudel *et al.*, 1988). The level of expression in brain was estimated to be about one-tenth that seen in skeletal muscle. The expression of the DMD gene in neuronal tissue may have direct consequences for the mental retardation seen in the patients but does not explain the variability across patients. The question will most likely be answered by the study of the normal function of the DMD gene product in neuronal cells.

THE DMD/BMD PROTEIN

The nucleotide sequence of the entire human skeletal muscle cDNA has been determined in parallel with the sequence of the mouse cardiac cDNA. Approximately 30% has been compared between both species, and both sequences are aligned in Fig. 8 (Hoffman *et al.*, 1987). The transcriptional orientation of the DMD gene was previously established as centromere to telomere of the X-chromosome short arm. Only one uninterrupted open reading frame was found in the cDNA sequence and agreed with this orientation. The human cDNA sequence is 88% homologous at the nucleotide level with the mouse cardiac muscle sequence, and the predicted amino acid sequences of both are 86% homologous. There were no deletions or insertions of nucleotides or encoded amino acids. Between the human and mouse sequences, most nucleotide differences that changed single amino acids were conserved with regard to the hydrophobicity or hydrophilicity of the residues. The hydropathicity

```
Mouse  I  AGAGTTATGCCTTCACACAGGCTGCTTATGTTGCCACCTCTGATTCCACACAGAGCCCCT
           S  Y  A  P  T  Q  A  A  Y  V  A  T  S  D  S  T  Q  S  P  Y
           ATCCTTCACAGCATTTGCAAGCTCCCAGAGACAAGCTCACTTGACAGTTCATTGATGGACA
           P  S  Q  N  L  E  A  P  R  D  K  S  L  D  S  S  L  N  K  T
           CGGAAGTAAATCTGGATAGTTACCAAACTGCTTTAGAAGAAGTACTTTCATGGCTTCTTT
           E  V  N  L  D  S  Y  Q  T  A  L  E  E  V  L  S  W  L  L  S
           CTGCCGAGGATACATTGGCAGCACAAGGAGAGATTTCAAATGATGTTGAAGAAGTGAAG
           A  E  D  T  L  R  A  Q  G  E  I  S  N  D  V  E  E  V  K  E
           AACAGTTTCATGCTCATGAGGGATTCATGATGGATCTGACATCTCATCAAGGACTTGTTG
           Q  F  M  A  H  E  G  P  M  M  D  L  T  S  H  Q  G  L  V  G
           GTAATGTTCTACAGTTAGGAAGTCAACTAGTTGGAAAAGGGAAATTATCAGAAGATGAAC
           N  V  L  Q  L  G  S  Q  L  V  G  K  G  K  L  S  E  D  E  E
           AAGCTGAAGTGCAAGAACAAATGAATCTCCTAAATTCAAGATGGGAATGTCTCAGGGTAG
           A  E  V  Q  E  Q  M  H  N  L  L  N  S  R  W  E  C  L  R  V  A
           CTAGCATGGAAAAACAAAGCAAATTACACAAAGTTCTAATGGATCTCCAGAATCAGAAAT
           S  M  E  K  Q  Q  S  K  L  H  K  V  L  M  D  L  Q  N  Q  K  L
           TAAAAGAACTAGATGACTGGTTAACAAAAACTGAAGAGAGAACTAAGAAAATGGAGGAAG
           K  E  L  D  D  W  L  T  K  T  E  E  R  T  K  K  M  E  K  E

Mouse      AGCCCTTTGGGACCTGATCTTGAAGATCTAAAATGCCAAGTACAACAACATAAGGTGCTT
           P  F  G  P  D  L  E  D  L  K  C  Q  V  Q  Q  H  K  V  L
                                            I  Q  Q  H  K  V  L
Human  I                                   ACAACAACATAAGGTGCTT

             *              *
           CAAGAACGATCTAGAACAAGAACAGGTCAGGGTCAACTCGCTCACTCACATGGTAGTAGTG
           Q  E  D  L  E  Q  E  Q  V  R  V  N  S  L  T  H  M  V  V  V
           Q  E  D  L  E  Q  E  Q  V  R  V  N  S  L  T  H  M  V  V  V
           CAAGAACGATCTAGAACAAGAACAAGTCAGGGTCAATTCTCTCACTCACATGTTGGTGGTA

             *        *        *      *      *
           GTTGATGAATCCAGCGGTGATCATCGAACAGCTGCTTTGGAAGAACAACTTAAGGTACTG
           V  D  E  S  S  G  D  H  A  T  A  A  L  E  E  Q  L  K  V  L
           V  D  E  S  S  G  D  H  A  T  A  A  L  E  E  Q  L  K  V  L
           GTTGATGAATCCAGTGGAGATCACGCAACTGCTGCTTTGGAAGAACAACTTAAGGTATTG

           GCAGATCGATGGGCAAATATCTGCAGATGGACTGAAGACCTGGATTGTTTTTTACAAGAT
           G  D  R  W  A  N  I  C  R  W  T  E  D  K  W  [V V]  L  Q  D
           G  D  R  W  A  N  I  C  R  W  T  E  D  R  W  [W L]  K  L  Q
           GCAGAGATCGATGGGCAAACATCTGTAGATGGCACAGAACACCGCTGGGTTCTTTTACAAGAC

             *        ***
           ATTCTTCTAAAATGCCAGCATTTTACTGAAGAACAGTGCCTTTTTAGTACATGGCTTTCA
           I  L  L  K  W  Q  [N F]  T  E  E  Q  C  L  F  S  [T]  W  L  S
           I  L  L  K  W  Q  [R L]  T  E  E  Q  C  L  F  S  [A]  W  L  S
           ATCCTTCTCAAATGCCAACGTCTTACTGAAGAACAGTGCCTTTTTAGTGCATGGCTTTCA

           GAAAAAGAAGATGCAATGAAGAACATTCAGACAAGTGGCTTTAAAGATCAAAATGAAATG
           E  K  E  D  A  [M K N I]  Q  T  S  G  F  K  D  Q  N  E  M
           E  K  E  D  A  [V N K I H]  T  T  G  F  K  D  Q  N  E  M
           GAAAAAGAAGATGCAGTGAACAAGAATTCACACAACTGGCTTTAAAGATCAAAATGAAATG

             **       *
           ATGTCAAGTCTTCACAAAAATATCTACTTTAAAAATAGATCTAGAAAGAAAAAGCCAACC
           [M S S L]  [R K I S T L K]  [I]  D  L  E  K  K  K  [F T]
           [L S S L K]  [L A V L K A]  [D]  L  E  K  K  K  [Q S]
           TTATCAAGTCTTCAAAAACTGGCCGTTTTAAAAGCGGATCTAGAAAAGAAAAACAATCC

           ATGCAAAAACTAAGTTCACTCAATCAAGATCTACTTTCGGCCACTGAAAAATAAGTCAGTG
           M  [E]  K  L  [S S]  L  N  Q  D  L  L  S  [A]  L  K  N  K  S  V
           M  [G]  K  L  [Y]  S  L  K  Q  D  L  L  S  [V]  A  R  E  K  L  Q  T  I  F
           ATGGGCAAACTGTATTCACTCAAACAAGATCTTCTTCAACACTGAAGAATAAGTCAGTG

             *          *  ***      *      **
           ACTCAAAAGATGAAATCTGGATGAAAACTTTGCACAACGTTGGGCACAATTTAACCCAA
           T  Q  K  [N E]  W  N  [E N]  F  A  Q  R  W  D  N  L  [T]  Q
           T  Q  K  [T E A]  W  [L]  D  N  F  A  [R C]  W  D  N  L  [V]  Q
           ACCCAGAAGACACAGAAGCTGGCTCGGATAACTTTGCCCGGTGTTGGGATAATTTAGTCCAA

           AAACTTGAAAAGAGTTCAGCACAAATTTCACAGGCTGTCACCACCACTCAACCATTCCTA
           K  L  E  K  S  [S]  A  Q  I  S  Q  A  V  T  T  T  Q  P  [V L]
           K  L  E  K  S  [T]  A  Q  I  S  Q  A  V  T  T  T  Q  P  [S L]
           AAACTTGAAAAGAGTACAGCACAAATTTCACAGGCTGTCACCACCACTCAGCCATCACTA

             *        **
           ACACAGACAACTGTAATGGAAACAACTGTACATGTGACCAACAAGGGAACAAATCATGGTA
           T  Q  T  T  V  M  E  T  T  V  [T H]  V  T  T  R  E  Q  I  [H V]
           T  Q  T  T  V  M  E  T  T  V  [T I]  V  T  T  R  E  Q  I  [N V]
           ACACAGACAACTGTAATGGAAACAuTAACTACGTGACCACAAGGGAACAGATCAuTGGTA

             *          ***            *
           AAACATGCCCAAGAGCAACTTCCACCACCACCTCCTCAAAAGAAGAGGCAGATAAACTGTG
           K  H  A  Q  E  E  L  P  P  P  P  P  P  Q  K  K  R  Q  I  T  V
           K  H  A  Q  E  E  L  P  P  P  P  P  Q  K  K  R  Q  I  T  V
           AAGCACTGCCCAAGAGCAACTTCCACCACCACCTCCCCAAAAGAAGAGGCAGATTACTGTG
```

```
             **             *
           GATTCTGAACTCAGGAAAAGGTTGGATGTCGATATAACTGAACTTCACGTTTGGATTACT
           D  S  E  [L R]  E  K  R  L  D  V  D  I  T  E  L  N  S  W  I  T
           D  S  E  [I]  R  E  K  R  L  D  V  D  I  T  E  L  N  S  W  I  T
           GATTCTGAAATTAGGAAAAGGTTGGATGTTGATATAACTGAACTTCACAGCTGGATTACT

             *      *        *       **    *
           CGTTCAGAAGCTGTATTACAGAGTTCTGAATTTGCAGTCTATCGAAAAGAAGGCAACATC
           R  S  E  A  V  L  Q  S  [S K F A]  [V Y]  R  K  E  G  N  [N]
           R  S  E  A  V  L  Q  S  [P E F A]  [I]  P  R  K  E  G  N  [P]
           CGCTCAGAAGCTCTGTTGCAGACTCCTGAATTTGCAATCTTTCGGAAGCAAGGCAACTTC

             **
           TCAGACTTGCAAGAAAAAGTCAATGCCATAGCACGAGAAAAAGCAGAGAAGTTCAGAAAA
           S  D  L  [Q]  E  K  V  N  A  I  [A]  R  E  K  A  E  K  F  R  K
           S  D  L  [K]  E  K  V  N  A  I  [E]  R  E  K  A  E  K  F  R  K
           TCAGACTTAAAAGAAAAAGTCAATGCCATAGAGCGAGAAAAAGCTGAAGAGTTCAGAAAA

             **
           CTGCAAGATGCCAGCAGATCAGCTCAGGCCCTGGTGGAACAGATGGCAAATGAGGGTGTT
           L  Q  D  A  S  R  S  A  Q  A  L  V  E  Q  M  [A]  N  E  G  V
           L  Q  D  A  S  R  S  A  Q  A  L  V  E  Q  M  [V]  N  E  G  V
           CTGCAAGATGCCAGCAGATCAGCTCAGGCCCTGGTGGAACAGATGGTGAATGAGGGTGTT

             *    *      *    *        *
           AATGCTGAAAGTATCAGACAAGCTTCAGAACAACTGAACAGCCGGTGGACAGAATTCTGC
           N  A  E  S  I  [K]  Q  A  S  E  Q  L  N  S  R  W  [T]  E  F  C
           N  A  D  S  I  [K]  Q  A  S  E  Q  L  N  S  R  W  [I]  E  F  C
           AATGCAGATAGCATCAAACAAGCCTCAGAACAACTGAACAGCCGGTGGATCGAATTCTGC

             *      *
           CAATTGCTGAGTGAGAGAGTTAACTGGCTAGAGTATCAAAACCAACATCATTAGTCTTTTAT
           Q  L  L  S  E  R  [V]  N  W  L  E  Y  Q  [T N]  I  I  [T F]  Y
           Q  L  L  S  E  R  [L]  N  W  L  E  Y  Q  [N N]  I  [A]  F  Y
           CAGTTGCTAAGTGAGAGCTTAACTGGCTGGAGTATCAGAACAACATCATCGCTTTCTAT

           AATCAGCTACAACAATTGGACGAGATGACAACTACTGCCGAAAACTTGTTGAAAACCCAG
           N  Q  L  Q  Q  L  E  Q  M  T  T  T  A  E  N  [L]  L  K  T  Q
           N  Q  L  Q  Q  L  E  Q  M  T  T  T  A  E  N  [W]  L  K  L  Q
           AATCAGCTACAACAATTGGAGCAGATGACAACTACTGCTGAAAACTGGTTGAAAATCCAA

             * *
           TCTACCACCCTATACAGAGCCAACAGCAATTAAAAGCCAGTTAAAAATTTGTAAGGATGAA
           S  T  T  [L]  S  E  P  T  A  I  K  S  Q  L  K  I  C  K  D  E
           P  T  T  [P]  S  E  P  T  A  I  K  S  Q  L  K  I  C  K  D  E
           CCCACCACCCCATCAGAGCCAACAGCAATTAAAAGTCAGTTAAAAATTTGTAAGGATGAA

             **
           GTCAACAGATTGTCAGCTCTTCAGCCTCAAATTGAGCAATTAAAAATTCAGAGTCTACAA
           V  N  R  L  S  [A]  L  Q  P  Q  I  E  [K]  L  K  I  Q  S  [L Q]
           V  N  R  L  S  [C]  L  Q  P  Q  I  E  [R]  L  K  I  Q  S  [I A]
           GTCAACCGGCTATCAGGTCTTCAACCTCAAATTGAACGATTAAAAATTCAAAGCATAGCC

           CTGAAAGAAAAAGGACAGGGGCCAATGTTTCTGGATGCAGATTTGTGGCCTTTACTAAT
           L  K  E  K  G  Q  G  P  M  F  L  D  A  D  F  V  A  F  T  N
           L  K  E  K  G  Q  G  P  M  F  L  D  A  D  F  V  A  F  T  N
           CTGAAAGAGAAAGGACAAGGACCCATGTTCCTGGATGCAGACTTTGTGGCCTTTACAAAT

           CATTTTAACCACATCTTTGATGGTGTGAGGGCCAAAGAGAAAGAGCTACAGACAATATTT
           H  F  [N H I]  F  D  G  V  [R]  A  K  E  K  E  L  Q  T  I  F
           H  F  [K Q V]  S  D  V  Q  A  R  E  K  E  L  Q  T  I  F
           CATTTAAGCAAGTCTTTTCGATGTGCAGGCCAGAGAGAAAAAGGAGCTACAGACAATATTT

           GACACTTTACCACCAATGCGCTATCAGGAGACAATGAGTAGCATCAGGACCGTGGATCCAG
           D  T  L  P  P  M  R  Y  Q  E  T  M  S  [S]  I  R  T  [W T]  Q
           D  T  L  P  P  M  R  Y  Q  E  T  M  S  [A]  I  R  T  [W]  V  Q
           GACACTTTGCCACCAATGCGCTATCAGGAGACCATGAGTGCCATCAGGACAGTGGCTCCAG

           CAGTCAGAAAGCAAACTCTCTGTACCTTATCTTAGTGTTACTGAATATGAAATAATGGAG
           Q  S  K  [S K L S]  [V P]  Y  L  S  V  T  [P V L]
           Q  S  E  T  K  L  S  [I P]  Q  L  S  V  T  [D]  Y  E  I  M  E
           CAGTCAGAAACCAAACTCTCCATACCTCAACTTAGTGTCACCGACTATGAAATCATGGAG

           GAGAGACTCGGGAAATTACAAGGCTCTGCAAAGTTCTTTGAAAGAGCAACAAAATGGCTTC
           [E R L G K L Q A L Q S S L K E Q Q N G F]
           [Q R L G K L Q A L Q S S L K E Q Q S G L]
           CAGAGACTCGGGGAATTGCAGGCTTTACAAAGTTCTCTGCAAGAGCAAAAGTGGCCTTA

             *      ***      *          **
           AACTACTGTAGTGACACTGTGAAGGAGATGGCCAAGAAAGCACCTTCAGAAATATGCCAG
           [H Y L S D T V K E N A K K A P S E I C Q]
           [Y Y L S T T V K E N S K K A P S E I S R]
           TGTTATCTCACCACTACTGTGAAGGAGATGTCGAAGAAAGCGCCCTCTGAAATTAGCCGC
```

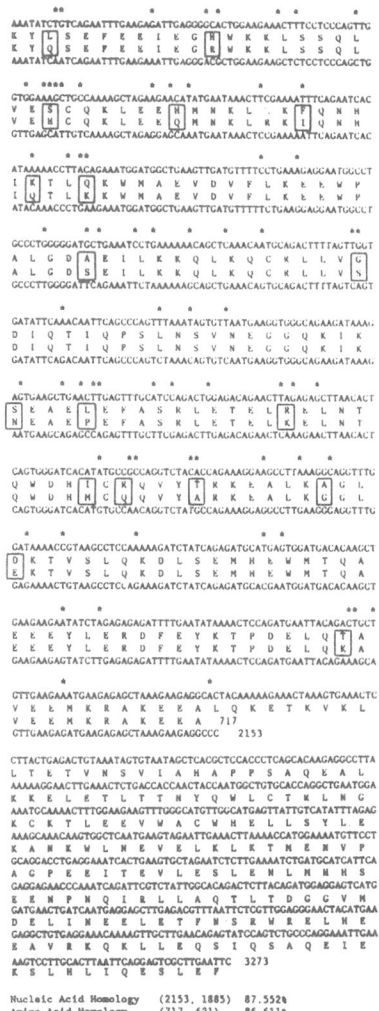

Fig. 8.   Nucleotide and predicted amino acid sequences of mouse and human cDNAs for a portion of the DMD gene. The cDNAs were subcloned in plasmid vectors (Stratagene Bluescript) and subjected to either chemical (Maxam and Gilbert, 1977) or chain-terminating (Sanger *et al.*, 1977) sequencing methods. Clones were sequenced on both strands. Sequence translations and alignments were done on the Bionet resource, Intelligenetics. Differences between the mouse and human DNA sequences are indicated by asterisks, while amino acid differences are boxed.

plots indicate almost complete identity between the human and mouse sequences, with predominately hydrophilic, α-helix-rich domains (Chou and Fasman, 1974; Bionet @PPEP; U. Wis. $PEP-PLOT).

Both the human and mouse predicted proteins have many charged amino acids (33% E + R + L + K) among hydrophobic residues. The sequence has short stretches of homology (seven or eight residues) with α-helices seen in structural muscle proteins such as the myosin heavy chains, tropomyosin, troponin T, desmin, keratin, laminin, and apolipoproteins B and C (Bionet @IFIND of NBRF protein database). These proteins contain a repeat of seven amino acids (a-b-c-d-e-f-g) best documented in the coiled-coil portions of the structural proteins (Cohen and Parry, 1986; McLachlin and Karn, 1982; Strehler *et al.*, 1986). Hydrophobic residues are usually located at residues a and d, where they interact between the two strands of the protein to form coiled-coils. The charged residues are concentrated at positions b, c, and f, where they would function at the helix surface. The seven-amino acid repeat is arranged in a larger domain of 28 amino acids that can be separated by "skip" residues. The amino acid sequence found in the DMD gene contains the helix-breaking residues proline and glycine, which is more characteristic of the hinge region of myosin rather than the uninterrupted rod portion (Lu and Wong, 1985). The high level of conservation between the human and mouse sequences may indicate highly conserved interactions with other muscle structural proteins that are part of the contractile apparatus. The complete 14-kb cDNA representation of the DMD gene has been recently isolated and the nucleotide sequence determined (Koenig *et al.*, 1987, 1988). The predicted protein product dystrophin has 3685 encoded amino acids and is organized into four domains. The N-terminal domain (240 amino acids) is similar to the actin binding portion of α-actinin. The large second domain consists of 25 triple helical segments in succession that have similarity to the rod-shaped domains of spectrin and α-actinin (Davidson and Critchley, 1988). The third domain is a cysteine-rich segment with similarity to the C-terminal domain of α-actinin while the last domain of 420 amino acids has no similarity to known protein sequences. Thus, dystrophin is most likely a member of a superfamily of flexible rod-shaped cytoskeletal proteins that includes spectrin and α-actinin (Koenig *et al.*, 1988).

Polyclonal antibodies raised against two different N-terminal domains of the protein product dystrophin recognize an approximately 400-kd protein in skeletal, smooth, and cardiac muscle and brain (Hoffman *et al.*, 1987b). The protein dystrophin has been localized to the muscle plasma membrane and t-tubules by subcellular fractionation and immunofluorescence and has been shown to be missing in DMD and mdx muscle samples (Hoffman *et al.*, 1987*b*, *c*; Sugita *et al.*, 1988). Dystrophin was found to be absent in most DMD-affected individuals and in mdx mice, yet BMD patients were found to have altered size proteins (Hoffman *et al.*, 1988). This result confirms the open reading frame hypothesis for the clinical difference between DMD and BMD patients bearing partial gene deletions (see pp. 85–86, and Monaco *et al.*, 1988).

FUTURE PROSPECTS

The DMD locus is unusually large and predicts a large protein. Insights into the structure and function of the DMD protein have emerged from the complete sequence of the cDNA and the generation of antibodies to the predicted peptide sequence. One of the major questions relating to the study of such a devastating disorder is whether therapy will result. The cloning of the DMD gene and the characterization of the protein should be steps in this direction. Possibly these basic facts may make intervention in the progression of the phenotype something to look forward to in the future. At the moment one can only hope for this to become a reality. The huge size of the DMD locus and the resultant high mutational frequency will make DMD a difficult but not impossible gene to manipulate.

ACKNOWLEDGMENTS.   The authors would like to thank all the scientists and clinicians who have contributed to the cloning of the Duchenne gene, but a special thanks are reserved for the members of the Kunkel laboratory, Bill Middlesworth, Chris Feener, Corlee Bertelson, Eric Hoffman, and Michel Koenig, who have contributed hard work, data, and ideas toward the completion of this project. We would also like to thank G. J. van Ommen, Margit Burmeister, and Ronald Worton for communicating unpublished information. A special thanks is also given to Samuel A. Latt, in whose laboratory the early work on this project was initiated. Much of this review fulfilled the Ph.D. thesis requirements of A.P.M. at Harvard University. This work was supported by the Muscular Dystrophy Association, the National Institutes of Health (NS23740), and the Howard Hughes Medical Institute.

REFERENCES

Aldridge, J., Kunkel, L., Bruns, G., Tantravahi, U., Lalande, M., Brewster, T., and Moreau, E., 1984, A strategy to reveal high frequency RFLPs along the human X chromosome, *Am. J. Hum. Genet.* **36**:546–564.

Appel, S. H., and Roses, A. D., 1983, The muscular dystrophies, in: *The Metabolic Basis of Inherited Disease* (J. B. Stanbury, ed.), pp. 1470–1495, McGraw-Hill, New York.

Baehner, R. L., Kunkel, L. M., Monaco, A. P., Haines, J. L., Conneally, P. M., Palmer, C., Heerema, N., and Orkin, S. H., 1986, DNA linkage analysis of X-chromosome-linked chronic granulomatous disease, *Proc. Natl. Acad. Sci. USA* **83**:3398–3401.

Bakker, E., Hofker, M. H., Goor, N., Mandel, J. L., Wrogemann, K., Davies, K. E., Kunkel, L. M., Willard, H. F., Fenton, W. A., Sandkuyl, L., van Ommen, G.-J. B., and Pearson, P. L., 1985, Prenatal diagnosis and carrier detection of Duchenne muscular dystrophy with closely linked RFLPs, *Lancet* **1**:655–658.

Bakker, E., Van Broeckhoven, Ch., Bonten, E. J., van de Vooren, M. J., Veenema, H., Van Hul, W., Van Ommen, G. J. B., Vandenberghe, A., and Pearson, P. L., 1987, Germline mosaicism and Duchenne muscular dystrophy mutations, *Nature* **329**:554–556.

Bartley, J. A., Patil, S., Davenport, S., Goldstein, D., and Pickens, J., 1986, Duchenne muscular dystrophy, glycerol kinase deficiency, and adrenal insufficiency associated with an Xp21 interstitial deletion, *J. Pediatr.* **108**:189–192.

Bender, W., Arkam, M., Karch, F., Beachy, P. A., Peifer, M., Spierer, P., Lewis, E. B., and Hogness, D. S., 1983, Molecular genetics of the bithorax complex in *Drosophila melanogaster, Science* **221**:23–29.

Benton, W. D., and Davis, R. W., 1977, Screening lambda-gt recombinant clones by hybridization to single plaques *in situ, Science* **196**:180–182.

Bertelson, C. J., Bartley, J. A., Monaco, A. P., Colletti-Feener, C., Fischbeck, K., and Kunkel, L. M., 1986, Localization of Xp21 meiotic exchange points in DMD families, *J. Med. Genet.* **23**:531–537.

Bertelson, C. J., Pogo, A. O., Chauduri, A., Marsh, W. L., Redman, C. M., Banerjee, D., Symmans, W. A., Simon, T., Frey, D., and Kunkel, L. M., 1988, Localization of the McLeod locus (XK) within Xp21 by deletion analysis, *Am. J. Hum. Genet.* **42**:703–711.

Blau, H. M., Webster, C., and Pavlath, G. K., 1983, Defective myoblasts identified in Duchenne muscular dystrophy, *Proc. Natl. Acad. Sci. USA* **80**:4856–4860.

Bolivar, F., Rodriguez, R. L., Greene, P. J., Betlach, M. C., Heyneker, H. L., Boyer, H. W., Crosa, H. J., and Falkow, S., 1977, Construction and characteristics of new cloning vehicles. II. A multipurpose cloning system, *Gene* **2**:95–113.

Botstein, D., White, R. L., Skolnick, M., and Davis, R. W., 1980, Construction of a genetic linkage map in man using restriction fragment length polymorphisms, *Am. J. Hum. Genet.* **32:**314–331.

Boyd, Y., and Buckle, V. J., 1986, Cytogenetic heterogeneity of translocations associated with Duchenne muscular dystrophy, *Clin. Genet.* **29:**108–115.

Boyd, Y., Munro, E., Ray, P., Worton, R., Monaco, A., Kunkel, L. M., and Craig, I., 1987, Molecular heterogeneity of translocations associated with muscular dystrophy, *Clin. Genet.* **31:**265–272.

Breitbart, R. E., Nguyen, H. T., Medford, R. M., Destree, A. T., Mahdavi, V., and Nadal-Ginard, B., 1985, Intricate combinatorial patterns of exon splicing generate multiple regulated troponin T isoforms, *Cell* **41:**67–82.

Britten, R. J., and Kohne, D. E., 1968, Repeated sequences in DNA, *Science* **161:**529–540.

Brooke, M. H., Fenichel, G. M., Griggs, R. C., Mendell, J. R., Moxley, R., Miller, J. P., Province, M. A., and the CIDD Group, 1983, Clinical investigations in Duchenne muscular dystrophy: 2. Determination of the "power" of therapeutic trials based on the natural history, *Muscle Nerve* **6:**91–103.

Brown, C. S., Thomas, N. S. T., Sarfarazi, M., Davies, K. E., Kunkel, L., Kingston, H. M., Shaw, D. J., and Harper, P. S., 1985, Genetic linkage relationships of seven DNA probes with Duchenne and Becker muscular dystrophy, *Hum. Genet.* **71:**62–74.

Brown, W. R. A., and Bird, A. P., 1986, Long range restriction site mapping of mammalian genomic DNA, *Nature* **322:**477–481.

Burghes, A. H. M., Logan, C., Hu, X., Belfall, B., Worton, R. G., and Ray, P. N., 1987, A cDNA clone from the Duchenne/Becker muscular dystrophy gene, *Nature* **328:**434–437.

Burmeister, M., and Lehrach, H., 1986, Long-range restriction map around the Duchenne muscular dystrophy gene, *Nature* **324:**582–585.

Carle, G. F., Frank, M., and Olson, M. V., 1986, Electrophoretic separations of large DNA molecules by periodic inversion of the electric field, *Science* **4:**65–68.

Carpenter, S., and Karpati, G., 1979, Duchenne muscular dystrophy. Plasma membrane loss initiates muscle cell necrosis unless it is repaired, *Brain* **102:**147–161.

Chamberlain, J. S., Pearlman, J. A., Muzny, D. M., Gibbs, R. A., Ranier, J. E., Reeves, A. A., and Caskey, C. T., 1988, Expression of the murine Duchenne muscular dystrophy gene in muscle and brain, *Science* **239:**1416–1418.

Chou, P. Y., and Fasman, G. D., 1974, Prediction of protein conformation, *Biochemistry* **13:**222–245.

Cohen, C., and Parry, D. A. D., 1986, α-Helical coiled-coils—A widespread motif in proteins, *Trends Biochem. Sci.* **11:**1–4.

Cullen, M. J., and Fulthorpe, J. J., 1975, Stages in fibre breakdown in Duchenne muscular dystrophy: An electron-microscopic study, *J. Neurol. Sci.* **24:**179–200.

Darras, B. T., and Francke, U., 1987, A partial deletion of the muscular dystrophy gene transmitted twice by an unaffected male, *Nature* **329:**556–558.

Davidson, M. D., and Critchley, D. R., 1988, α-Actinins and the DMD protein contain spectrin-like repeats, *Cell* **52:**159–160.

Davies, K. E., Young, B. D., Elles, R. G., Hill, M. E., and Williamson, R., 1981, Cloning of a representative genomic library of the human X chromosome after sorting by flow cytometry, *Nature* **293:**374–376.

Davies, K. E., Pearson, P. L., Harper, P. S., Murray, J. M., O'Brien, T., Sarfarazzi, M., and Williamson, R., 1983, Linkage analysis of two cloned DNA sequences flanking the Duchenne muscular dystrophy locus on the short arm of the human X chromosome, *Nucleic Acids Res.* **11**:2303–2312.

DeMartinville, B., Kunkel, L. M., Bruns, G., Morle, F., Koenig, M., Mandel, J. L., Horwich, A., Latt, S. A., Gusella, J. F., Housman, D., and Francke, U., 1985, Localization of DNA sequences in the region Xp21 of the human X chromosome: Search for molecular markers close to the Duchenne muscular dystrophy locus, *Am. J. Hum. Genet.* **37**:235–249.

Dorkins, H., Junien, C., Mandel, J. L., Wrogemann, K., Moison, J. P., Martinez, M., Old, J. M., Bundey, S., Schwartz, M., Carpenter, N., Hill, D., Lindlof, M., de la Chapelle, A., Pearson, P. L., and Davies, K. E., 1985, Segregation analysis of a marker localised on Xp21.2–Xp21.3 in Duchenne and Becker muscular dystrophy families, *Hum. Genet.* **71**:103–107.

Dubowitz, V., 1985, Muscular dystrophies, in: *Muscle Biopsy, A Practical Approach*, Tindall, London.

Emery, A. E. H., and Holloway, S., 1977, Use of normal daughters' and sisters' creatine kinase levels in estimating heterozygosity in Duchenne muscular dystrophy, *Hum. Hered.* **27**:118–126.

Fadda, S., Mochi, M., Roncuzzi, L., Sangiori, S., Sbarra, D., Katz, M., and Romeo, G., 1985, Definitive localization of Becker muscular dystrophy in Xp by linkage to a cluster of DNA polymorphisms (DXS43 and DXS9), *Hum. Genet.* **71**:33–36.

Fingerman, E., Campisi, J., and Pardee, A. B., 1984, Defective Ca^{2+} metabolism in Duchenne muscular dystrophy: Effects on cellular and viral growth, *Proc. Natl. Acad. Sci. USA* **81**:7617–7621.

Fischbeck, K. H., Ritter, A. W., Tirschwell, D. L., Kunkel, L. M., Bertelson, C. J., Monaco, A. P., Hejtmancik, J. F., Boehm, C., Ionasescu, V., Ionasescu, R., Pericak-Vance, M., Kandt, R., and Roses, A. D., 1986, Recombination with pERT87 (DXS164) in families with X-linked muscular dystrophy, *Lancet* **2**:104.

Francke, U., Ochs, H. D., de Martinville, B., Giacalone, J., Lindgren, V., Disteche, C. M., Pagon, R. A., Hofker, M. H., van Ommen, G.-J. B., Pearson, P. L., and Wedgwood, R. J., 1985, Minor Xp21 chromosome deletion in a male associated with expression of Duchenne muscular dystrophy, chronic granulomatous disease, retinitis pigmentosa, and McLeod syndrome, *Am. J. Hum. Genet.* **37**:250–267.

Francke, U., Harper, J. F., Darras, B. T., Cowan, J. M., McCabe, E. R. B., Kohlschutter, A., Seltzer, W. K., Saito, F., Goto, J., Harpey, J. P., and Wise, J. E., 1987, Congenital adrenal hypoplasia, myopathy and glycerol kinase deficiency: Molecular genetic evidence for deletions, *Am. J. Hum. Genet.* **40**:212–227.

Fryns, J. P., Kleczkowska, A., Petit, P., and van den Berghe, H., 1982, Fertility in patients with X-chromosome deletions, *Clin. Genet.* **22**:76–79.

Goodfellow, P. N., Davies, K. E., and Ropers, H. H., 1985, Report of the committee on the genetic constitution of the X and Y chromosomes, *Cytogenet. Cell Genet.* **40**:296–352.

Greenstein, R. M., Reardon, M. P., Chan, T. S., Middleton, A. B., Mulivor, R. A., Greene, A. E., and Coriell, L. L., 1980, An (X;11) translocation in a girl with Duchenne muscular dystrophy, *Cytogenet. Cell. Genet.* **27**:268.

Gubler, U., and Hoffman, B. J., 1983, A very simple and very efficient method for generating cDNA libraries, *Gene* **25**:263–269.

Hart, K. A., Hodgson, S., Walker, A., Cole, C. G., Johnson, L., Dubowitz, V., and Bobrow, M., 1987*a*, DNA deletions in mild and severe Becker muscular dystrophy, *Hum. Genet.* **75**:281–285.

Hart, K. A., Monaco, A. P., Kunkel, L. M., and Bobrow, M., 1987*b*, A small deletion in the Duchenne/Becker muscular dystrophy locus—A functionally important region? *Hum. Genet.* **77**:88–91.

Hoffman, E. P., Monaco, A. P., Feener, C. C., and Kunkel, L. M., 1987*a*, Conservation of the Duchenne muscular dystrophy gene in mice and humans, *Science* **238**:347–350.

Hoffman, E. P., Brown, R. H., Jr., and Kunkel, L. M., 1987*b*, Dystrophin: The protein product of the Duchenne muscular dystrophy locus, *Cell* **51**:919–928.

Hoffman, E. P., Knudson, C. M., Campbell, K. P., and Kunkel, L. M., 1987*c*, Subcellular fractionation of dystrophin to the triads of skeletal muscle, *Nature* **330**:754–758.

Hoffman, E. P., Fishbeck, K., Brown, R. H., Johnson, M., Medori, R., Loike, J. D., Harris, J. B., Waterston, R., Brooke, M., Specht, L., Kupsky, W., Chamberlain, J., Caskey, C. T., Shapiro, F., and Kunkel, L. M., 1988, Dystrophin quality and quantity determines the clinical severity of Duchenne/Becker muscular dystrophies, *N. Engl. J. Med.* (in press).

Hofker, M. H., Wapenaar, M. C., Coor, N., Bakker, E., van Ommen, G. J. B., and Pearson, P. L., 1985, Isolation of probes detecting restriction fragment length polymorphisms from X-chromosome specific libraries: Potential use for diagnosis of Duchenne muscular dystrophy, *Hum. Genet.* **70**:148–156.

Hu, D. H., Kimura, S., and Maruyama, K., 1986, Sodium dodecyl sulphate gel electrophoresis studies of connectin-like high molecular weight proteins of various types of vertebrate and invertebrate muscles, *J. Biochem.* **99**:1485–1492.

Huynh, T., Young, R. A., and Davis, R. W., 1985, Constructing and screening cDNA libraries in lambda gt10 and gt11, in: *DNA Cloning: A Practical Approach* (D. M. Glover, ed.), pp. 49–78, Oxford, England.

Jacobs, P. A., Hunt, P. A., Mayer, M., and Bart, R. D., 1981, Duchenne muscular dystrophy (DMD) in a female with an X/autosome translocation: Further evidence that the DMD locus is in Xp21, *Am. J. Hum. Genet.* **33**:513–518.

Kan, Y. W., and Dosy, A. M., 1978, Polymorphism of DNA sequence adjacent to human B-globin structural gene: Relationship to sickle mutation, *Proc. Natl. Acad. Sci. USA* **75**:5631–5635.

Kenwrick, S., Patterson, M., Speer, A., Fischbeck, K., and Davies, K., 1987, Molecular analysis of the Duchenne muscular dystrophy region using pulsed field gel electrophoresis, *Cell* **48**:351–357.

Kingston, H. M., Sarfarazi, M., Thomas, N. S. T., and Harper, P. S., 1984, Localization of the Becker muscular dystrophy gene on the short arm of the X chromosome by linkage to cloned DNA sequences, *Hum. Genet.* **67**:6–17.

Koenig, M., Hoffman, E. P., Bertelson, C. J., Monaco, A. P., Feener, C., and Kunkel, L. M., 1987, Complete cloning of the Duchenne muscular dystrophy (DMD) cDNA and preliminary genomic organization of the DMD gene in normal and affected individuals, *Cell* **50**:509–517.

Koenig, M., Monaco, A. P., and Kunkle, L. M., 1988, The complete sequence of dystrophin predicts a rod-shaped cytoskeletal protein, *Cell* **53**:219–228.

Kohne, D. E., Levinson, S. A., and Byers, M. J., 1977, Room temperature method for increasing the rate of DNA reassociation by many thousandfold: The phenol emulsion reassociation technique, *Biochemistry* **16**:5329–5341.

Kunkel, L. M., Tantravahi, U., Eisenhard, M., and Latt, S. A., 1982, Regional localization on the human X of DNA segments cloned from flow-sorted chromosomes, *Nucleic Acids Res.* **10**:1557–1578.

Kunkel, L. M., Lalande, M., Monaco, A. P., Flint, A., Middlesworth, W., and Latt, S. A., 1985a, Construction of a human X-chromosome-enriched phage library which facilitates analysis of specific loci, *Gene* **33**:251–258.

Kunkel, L. M., Monaco, A. P., Middlesworth, W., Ochs, H. D., and Latt, S. A., 1985b, Specific cloning of DNA fragments absent from the DNA of a male patient with an X chromosome deletion, *Proc. Natl. Acad. Sci. USA* **82**:4778–4782.

Kunkel, L. M., and co-authors, 1986, Analysis of deletions in the DNA of patients with Becker and Duchenne muscular dystrophy, *Nature* **322**:73–77.

Lamar, E. E., and Palmer, E., 1984, Y-encoded, species-specific DNA in mice: Evidence that the Y-chromosome exists in two polymorphic forms in inbred strains, *Cell* **37**:171–177.

Lange, K., Kunkel, L. M., Aldridge, J., and Latt, S. A., 1985, Accurate and super-accurate gene mapping, *Am. J. Hum. Genet.* **37**:853–867.

Locker, R. H., and Wild, D. J. C., 1986, A comparative study of high molecular weight proteins in various types of muscle across the animal kingdom, *J. Biochem.* **99**:1473–1484.

Lu, R. C., and Wong, A., 1985, The amino acid sequence and stability predictions of the hinge region in myosin subfragment 2, *J. Biol. Chem.* **260**:3456–3461.

Maxam, A. M., and Gilbert, W., 1977, A new method for sequencing DNA, *Proc. Natl. Acad. Sci. USA* **74**:560–564.

McLachlin, A. D., and Karn, J., 1982, Periodic charge distributions in the myosin rod amino acid sequence match cross-bridge spacings in muscle, *Nature* **299**:226–231.

Mokri, B., and Engel, A. G., 1975, Duchenne dystrophy: Electron microscopic findings pointing to a basic or early abnormality in the plasma membrane of the muscle fibers, *Neurology* **25**:1111–1120.

Monaco, A. P., and Kunkel, L. M., 1987, A giant locus for the Duchenne and Becker muscular dystrophy gene, *Trends Genet.* **3**:33–37.

Monaco, A. P., Bertelson, C. J., Middlesworth, W., Colletti, C. A., Aldridge, J., Fischbeck, K. H., Bartlett, R., Pericak-Vance, M. A., Roses, A. D., and Kunkel, L. M., 1985, Detection of deletions spanning the Duchenne muscular dystrophy locus using a tightly linked DNA segment, *Nature* **316**:842–845.

Monaco, A. P., Neve, R., Colletti-Feener, C., Bertelson, C. J., Kurnit, D. M., and Kunkel, L. M., 1986, Isolation of candidate cDNAs for portions of the Duchenne muscular dystrophy gene, *Nature* **323**:646–650.

Monaco, A. P., Bertelson, C. J., Colletti-Feener, C., and Kunkel, L. M., 1987, Localization and cloning of Xp21 deletion breakpoints involved in muscular dystrophy, *Hum. Genet.* **75**:221–227.

Monaco, A. P., Bertelson, C. J., Liechti-Gallati, S., Moser, H., and Kunkel, L. M.,

1988, An explanation for the phenotypic differences between patients bearing partial deletions of the DMD locus, *Genomics* **2**:90-95.

Moser, H., 1984, Duchenne muscular dystrophy: Pathogenetic aspects and genetic prevention, *Hum. Genet.* **66**:17-40.

Nudel, U., Robzyk K., and Yaffe, D., 1988, Expression of the putative Duchenne muscular dystrophy gene in differentiated myogenic cell cultures and in the brain, *Nature* **331**:635-638.

Orkin, S. H., and Kazazian, H. H., Jr., 1984, Mutation and polymorphism of the human B-globin gene and its surrounding DNA, *Annu. Rev. Genet.* **18**:131-171.

Perler, F., Efstratiadis, A., Lomedico, P., Gilbert, W., Kolodner, R., and Dodgson, J., 1980, The evolution of genes: The chicken preproinsulin gene, *Cell* **20**:555-566.

Ray, P. N., Belfall, B., Duff, C., Logan, C., Kean, V., Thompson, M. W., Sylvester, J. E., Gorski, J. L., Schmickel, R. D., and Worton, R. G., 1985, Cloning of the breakpoint of an X;21 translocation associated with Duchenne muscular dystrophy, *Nature* **318**:672-675.

Rosenfeld, M. G., Mermad, J.-J., Amara, S. G., Swanson, L. W., Sawchenko, P. E., Rivier, J., Vale, W., and Evans, R. M., 1983, Production of a novel neuropeptide encoded by the calcitonin gene via tissue specific RNA processing, *Nature* **304**:129-135.

Rowland, L. P., 1980, Biochemistry of muscle membranes in Duchenne muscular dystrophy, *Muscle Nerve* **3**:3-20.

Rozen, R., Fox, J., Fenton, W. A., Horwich, A. L., and Rosenberg, L. E., 1985, Gene deletion and restriction fragment length polymorphisms at the human ornithine transcarbamylase locus, *Nature* **313**:815-817.

Sanger, F., Nicklen, S., and Coulson, A. R., 1977, DNA sequencing with chain-terminating inhibitors, *Proc. Natl. Acad. Sci. USA* **74**:5463-5467.

Schwartz, D. C., and Cantor, C. R., 1984, Separation of yeast chromosome-sized DNAs by pulsed field gel electrophoresis, *Cell* **37**:67-75.

Singer, M. F., 1982, SINEs and LINEs: Highly repeated short and long interspersed sequences in mammalian genomes, *Cell* **28**:433-434.

Strehler, E. E., Strehler-Page, M.-A., Perriard, J.-C., Periasamy, M., and Nadal-Ginard, B., 1986, Complete nucleotide and encoded amino acid sequence of a mammalian myosin heavy chain gene, *J. Mol. Biol.* **190**:291-317.

Sugita, H., Arahata, K., Ishiguro, T., Suhara, Y., Tsukahara, T., Ishura, S., Eguchi, C., Nonaka, I., and Ozawa, E., 1988, Negative immunostaining of Duchenne muscular dystrophy (DMD) and mdx muscle surface membrane with antibody against synthetic peptide fragment predicted from DMD cDNA, *Proc. Japan Acad.* **64**:37-39.

Thomas, P. S., 1980, Hybridization of denatured RNA and small DNA fragments transferred to nitrocellulose, *Proc. Natl. Acad. Sci USA* **77**:5201-5205.

van Ommen, G.-J. B., Verkerk, J. M. H., Hofker, M. H., Monaco, A. P., Kunkel, L. M., Ray, P., Worton, R., Wieringa, B., Bakker, B., and Pearson, P. L., 1986, A physical map of 4 million bp around the Duchenne muscular dystrophy gene on the human X chromosome, *Cell* **47**:499-504.

Verellen-Dumoulin, Ch., Freund, M., DeMeyer, R., Laterre, Ch., Frederic, J., Thompson, M. W., Markovic, V. C., and Worton, R. G., 1984, Expression of an X-linked muscular dystrophy in a female due to translocation involving Xp21 and non-random inactivation of the normal X chromosome, *Hum. Genet.* **67:**115–119.

Webster, C., Filippi, B., Rinaldi, A., Mastropaolo, C., Tondi, M., Siniscalco, M., and Blau, H. M., 1986, The myoblast defect identified in Duchenne muscular dystrophy is not a primary expression of the DMD mutation, *Hum. Genet.* **74:**74–80.

Wetmur, J. G., and Davidson, N., 1968, Kinetics of renaturation of DNA, *J. Mol. Biol.* **31:**349–370.

Wieacker, P., Davies, K. E., Cooke, H. J., Pearson, P. L., Williamson, R., Bhattacharya, S., Zimmer, J., and Ropers, H. H., 1984, Toward a complete linkage map of the human X chromosome: Regional assignment of 16 cloned single-copy DNA sequences employing a panel of somatic cell hybrids, *Am. J. Hum. Genet.* **36:**265–276.

Wood, D. S., Sorenson, M. M., Eastwood, A. B., Charash, E., and Reuben, J. P., 1978, Duchenne dystrophy: Abnormal generation of tension and Ca+ + regulation in single skinned fibers, *Neurology* **28:**447–457.

Wood, D. S., Zeviani, M., Prelle, A., Bonilla, E., Salviati, G., Miranda, A. F., dMauro, S., and Rowland, L. P., 1987, Is nebulin the defective gene product in Duchenne muscular dystrophy? *N. Engl. J. Med.* **316:**107–108.

Worton, R. G., Duff, C., Sylvester, J. E., Schmickel, R. D., and Willard, H. F., 1984, Duchenne muscular dystrophy involving translocation of the DMD gene next to ribosomal RNA genes, *Science* **224:**1447–1449.

Yang, T. P., Patel, P. I., Chinault, A. C., Stout, J. T., Jackson, L. G., Hildebrand, B. M., and Caskey, C. T., 1984, Molecular evidence for new mutations at the HPRT locus in Lesch–Nyhan patients, *Nature* **310:**412–414.

Chapter 4

Trisomy 21
Molecular and Cytogenetic Studies of Nondisjunction

Gordon D. Stewart

University of Michigan Medical Center
Department of Pediatrics
Howard Hughes Medical Institute
Ann Arbor, Michigan 48109

Terry J. Hassold

Division of Medical Genetics
Emory University
Atlanta, Georgia 30322

David M. Kurnit

University of Michigan Medical Center
Departments of Pediatrics and Human Genetics
Howard Hughes Medical Institute
Ann Arbor, Michigan 48109

SCOPE OF THE PROBLEM

Chromosomal imbalance is the leading known cause of mental retardation (Smith and Berg, 1976), spontaneous abortion (Boué *et al.*, 1975; Carr and Gedeon, 1978; Hassold *et al.*, 1978), and congenital heart defects in man (Rowe and Uchida, 1961; Tandon and Edwards, 1973; Park *et al.*, 1977). Our understanding of nondisjunction is at a crossroads. Recent advances in molecular genetics and cytogenetics have afforded glimpses into the mechanisms of nondisjunction in man, and these advances will soon enable us to determine how and why nondisjunction for chromosome 21 occurs. This review has an agnostic, but optimistic, outlook. We feel that few fundamental questions relevant to nondisjunction for chromosome 21 have been resolved, but that the protocols and techniques required to obtain fundamental answers are at hand.

In this review, we summarize current information on the origin of nondisjunction for chromosome 21. For each of five outstanding problems relevant to these nondisjunction events, we discuss current hypotheses, experimental approaches, and the relevant molecular cytogenetic organization of chromosome 21. The first part of the review outlines these major unanswered problems that pertain to nondisjunction of chromosome 21. The middle part of the review summarizes current understanding of the molecular cytogenetic organization of chromosome 21 that is relevant to nondisjunction and presents results of a pilot study of trisomy 21. The last part of the review projects how recent advances in molecular genetics and cytogenetics will be applied to answer the fundamental problems outlined in the first part of the review.

PROBLEMS TO BE ADDRESSED

A. Complete and correct ascertainment of parental origin of nondisjunction.

B. The maternal age conundrum: Is the maternal age effect due to increased production of abnormal eggs or decreased destruction of abnormal embryos?

C. Identification of couples at high risk for trisomy 21 offspring.

D. Is there a correlation between crossing over and nondisjunction on chromosome 21?

E. The effect of the parental origin of trisomy on the phenotype of the conceptus.

Correct and Complete Ascertainment of Parental Origin of Nondisjunction

Studies of the parental origin of nondisjunction events involving chromosome 21 have been performed using cytogenetic polymorphisms on 21p, just above the centromere of chromosome 21. These polymorphisms, presumably resulting from quantitative variations in repeated DNA sequences in heterochromatin and ribosomal DNA (John and Miklos, 1979; Kurnit, 1979), can be detected visually using appropriate chromosome banding techniques. In informative families (i.e., when the parents' chromosome 21 homologues may be distinguished using these cytogenetic polymorphisms), it is possible to mark individual chromosome 21 homologues and to follow their segregation. Thus, in an informative family, it is possible to determine which parent was the source of the extra copy of chromosome 21. It is also possible to determine the stage of meiosis at which nondisjunction occurred, assuming that there has been no crossing over between the centromere and the cytogenetic marker on the short arm.

Based on this approach, more than 1000 Down syndrome individuals and parents have been studied over the past 15 years. (Bott et al., 1975; del Mazo et al., 1982; Jacobs and Mayer, 1981; Magenis et al., 1977; Mattei et al., 1980; Roberts and Callow, 1980; Wagenbicher et al., 1976; Mikkelsen et al., 1980; Houghton, 1981; Hansson and Mikkelsen, 1978; Juberg and Mowrey, 1983; Ayme et al., 1986). There is considerable variation among studies in the proportion of cases attributable to either parent, with the observed level of paternal nondisjunction ranging from 0% to 57%. Nevertheless, most studies agree that the majority of trisomy 21 results from nondisjunction at maternal meiosis I, but that one-third ensue from paternal errors or maternal meiosis II errors.

The cytogenetic studies have provided valuable information on the relative importance of different meiotic errors, but at least three technical problems limit their overall usefulness. First, analysis is based on subjective evaluation of the size and staining intensity of the chromosome variants, so that errors in assigning the parental origin of nondisjunction will occur. This is important, since even a small number of random errors may lead to erroneous conclusions (see below, discussion of maternal age) Second, cytogenetic polymorphisms are uninformative in a substantial fraction of families. Third, the chromosomal heteromorphisms on 21p are only on one side of the centromere, so that crossovers between the centromere

and the short-arm marker go undetected; such crossovers could con-
found attempts to distinguish whether nondisjunction is occurring
at first or second division. Additional objective DNA polymorphic
markers are needed to supplement the cytogenetic markers, to eliminate bias that might occur by selecting only families with distin-
guishable cytogenetic polymorphisms, and to sandwich the centromere between polymorphic markers on 21p and 21q. The worry
that bias may be inherent in such cytogenetic studies is suggested
by the recent assertion that cytogenetic heteromorphisms on the
short arm [e.g., the double nucleolus organizer (Jackson-Cook *et
al.*, 1985)] may be associated with an inherently increased risk for
nondisjunction. To circumvent these problems, DNA polymorphism
(Botstein *et al.*, 1980) and cytogenetic heteromorphism studies must
be employed jointly.

The Maternal Age Conundrum: Is the Maternal Age Effect due to Increased Production of Abnormal Eggs or Decreased Destruction of Abnormal Embryos?

The occurrence of trisomy 21 in offspring correlates strongly
with advanced maternal age: an exponential increase occurs in the
mid-30s, yielding a risk factor two orders of magnitude greater for
women in their mid-40s than for younger women (Penrose, 1933).
In contrast, advanced paternal age by itself does not appear to affect
the risk of having a child with trisomy 21 (Erickson, 1981; Hook *et
al.*, 1981; Hook and Regal, 1984).

The obvious hypothesis for the maternal age effect is that most
errors involving the numerical assortment of chromosome 21 occur
in eggs, with the error rate increasing as women age—an "older
egg" model. This model seems especially attractive given the finding
that Down syndrome resulting from translocation chromosomes
does not show this marked maternal age dependence (Kikuchi *et
al.*, 1969; Hamerton, 1971). However, studies using cytogenetic
polymorphisms to determine the parental origin of the extra chromosome 21 in Down syndrome subjects have not supported this
hypothesis. In studies of over 1000 Down syndrome families, about

70% of nondisjunction events involving chromosome 21 were maternal meiosis I errors, regardless of maternal age; thus, a maternal age effect was observed for both maternal and paternal errors. In contrast, the "older egg" model predicts that the proportion of maternal meiosis I errors will increase significantly with advancing maternal age.

These contradictions led to the "relaxed selection" hypothesis, which suggests the maternal age effect may ensue from an inability of older mothers to reject trisomy 21 conceptuses, resulting in a higher incidence of liveborn infants with Down syndrome (Ayme and Lippman-Hand, 1982; Stein et al., 1986). Recent studies in the mouse provide evidence that the maternal genotype can indeed affect the in utero survival of aneusomic conceptuses (Biddle et al., 1986; Vekemans and Trasler, 1985).

However, all the experimental evidence for an association between advanced maternal age and relaxed selection against trisomy 21 embryos is derived from analysis of cytogenetic heteromorphisms on 21p. These analyses are marred by the inability to determine parental origin in more than half of all couples, by the subjective nature of the cytogenetic polymorphism analysis, and by the use of markers on only one side (the short-arm side) of the centromere. Since trisomy 21 results most frequently from maternal meiosis I errors, both random technical errors and incomplete ascertainment will inflate the apparent proportion of all other errors (Langenbeck et al., 1976), thereby biasing the data against maternal meiosis I and the "older egg" model. Further, preliminary studies of 50 cases that use DNA polymorphisms to determine the parental origin of trisomy 21 do not demonstrate a clear-cut effect of maternal age on paternal nondisjunction errors (our data and personal communications from S. Antonarakis and N. Rudd). These last points are particularly relevant, since Carothers (1987) has demonstrated that an error rate as low as 8% in cytogenetic determinations of parental origin is sufficient to reconcile the published cytogenetic observations with an "older egg" model.

Taken together, the data do not clearly demonstrate whether the maternal age effect results from increased production of aneusomic eggs or decreased destruction of abnormal embryos: the lack of maternal age effect in translocation Down syndrome subjects supports the former hypothesis, and the cytogenetic heteromorphism data support the latter hypothesis. A large, coordinated study that utilizes both DNA-based polymorphisms on 21q and cytogenetic heteromorphisms on 21p to study nondisjunction of chromosome 21 is essential for the successful resolution of the maternal age conundrum.

Identification of Couples at High Risk for Trisomy 21 Offspring

Despite years of intensive study, advanced maternal age remains the only risk factor conclusively associated with nondisjunction in man. Cytogenetic and epidemiological studies have identified many candidate risk factors, including extrinsic factors such as cigarette smoking (Kline *et al.*, 1983), alcohol (Kaufman., 1983), maternal irradiation (Uchida, 1979), fertility drugs (Boué and Boué, 1973), oral contraceptives (Harlap *et al.*, 1979), and vaginal spermicides (Rothman, 1983; Strobino *et al.*, 1986), and intrinsic factors such as genes regulating nondisjunction (Alfi *et al.*, 1980), sharing of HLA antigens among parents (Mottironi, 1983), presence of antithyroid autoantibodies (Fialkow *et al.*, 1971; Flannery and Jackson-Cook, 1986), increased frequency of satellite associations between acrocentries (Jacobs and Mayer, 1981), and the presence of specific types of cytogenetic polymorphisms (e.g., Ford and Lester, 1978).

There are many possible explanations for the failure to identify important risk factors conclusively: it may be that researchers have failed to study the appropriate etiological agents or populations at risk. However, it may also be that the ability to detect an effect is limited by the study design. A major problem inherent in all studies to date is that the etiology of nondisjunction is inherently heterogeneous, as each of the four types of meiotic errors (maternal I, maternal II, paternal I, and paternal II) may have different genetic, environmental, and stochastic triggers. Thus, analysis should be partitioned for each class of meiotic error in a large, coordinated study that objectively determines the parental origin and stage of each error. Such a large, coordinated study could be used as a sensitive screen for risk factors that might be associated with each type of nondisjunction. In particular, analysis comparing each type of meiotic error against the others would provide internal controls.

Recently, several studies have used this approach in analyses of trisomy 21. For example, in a European collaborative study, epidemiological studies were combined with cytogenetic determinations of parental origin to identify a positive association between maternal irradiation and trisomy 21 of maternal origin (Ayme et al., 1986).

Two recent reports associated particular polymorphisms with an increased risk to have offspring with trisomy 21: (1) Jackson-Cooke et al. (1985) described an association between nondisjunction and a cytogenetic heteromorphic marker, the "double nucleolus-organizer region" (i.e., a doublet appearance of the darkly staining region on the short arm of human acrocentric chromosomes following silver staining of proteins associated with ribosomal RNA). No other group (Spinner et al., 1986; Hassold et al., 1987) has been able to confirm a high frequency of double nucleolus organizer variants in Down syndrome subjects and families. Given the high level of interest in this report, a number of studies are pending. Further, use of silver staining in a large-scale study that combines both cytogenetic and DNA markers will permit final resolution of this problem; again, this study will be more sensitive, as it will determine whether specific types of meiotic errors, presumably meiosis I errors, are associated with double nucleolus organizer regions. (2) Antonarakis et al. (1985) described a statistical association between nondisjunction and particular DNA polymorphisms on the proximal part of 21q. This conclusion remains problematic: these workers utilized probes on 21q that are at least 15 cm from the centromere of chromosome 21 (Tanzi et al., submitted; Antonarakis et al., 1986; Warren et al., 1987) and hence are unlikely to show tight linkage with any marker for nondisjunction associated directly with the centromere.

Further studies are needed to investigate the putative association between nondisjunction and maternal irradiation, double nucleolus organizing regions, specific DNA polymorphisms, and the other purported etiological agents. Nevertheless, the approach of using parental origin studies to search for such effects is sound. For

reasons discussed above, results obtained in studies using only cytogenetic heteromorphisms require reinvestigation using both DNA
polymorphisms on 21q and cytogenetic heteromorphisms on 21p.
Thus, future, larger scale studies should include a questionnaire designed to investigate whether maternal irradiation and a number of
other environmental agents are indeed associated with nondisjunction; in particular, such a study would also determine whether any
positive association correlates with errors occurring at specific
stages of meiosis in a given parent. Since current indications for
prenatal screening [advanced maternal age, decreased maternal
serum α-fetoprotein (Cuckle *et al.*, 1984; DiMaio *et al.*, 1987; Pueschel, 1987)] detect only a minority of subjects carrying Down syndrome fetuses, the development of new assays to detect important
risk factors would represent a major public health advance.

Is There a Correlation between Crossing Over and Nondisjunction on Chromosome 21?

In species with chiasmate meiosis, maintenance of pairing in
meiosis I requires at least one chiasma per bivalent. This suggests
that nondisjunction could ensue from reduction or elimination of
crossing over. In female *Drosophila,* the likelihood of nondisjunction
is increased both in several meiotic mutants that decrease recombination (Sandler, 1981) and in flies heterozygous for structural rear-
rangements that suppress crossing over (e.g., inversions) (Grell,
1979). X-chromosome nondisjunction is more likely to involve bi-
valents that have undergone zero or two exchanges than those with
one exchange (Merriam and Frost, 1964), suggesting that either failure to pair or "chromosome entanglement" (Bridges, 1916) due to
multiple exchanges can lead to aneusomy.

In mouse, S. A. Henderson and Edwards (1968) observed de-
clining chiasma frequencies and increased incidence of univalents
in aging mouse oocytes, and suggested that age-dependent trisomy
ensues from a reduction in crossing over. Since chiasma formation
occurs prenatally in the female, they elaborated a "production line"
model in which chiasma frequency was decreased in oocytes formed
later during development. Several studies have now confirmed the

age-related decrease in chiasmata and increase in univalents in the female mouse (Luthardt *et al.*, 1973; Polani and Jagiello, 1976; Speed, 1977), hamster (Sugawara and Mikamo, 1983), and human (Luthardt, 1977). Jagiello and Fang (1979) reported a lower chiasma frequency among mouse oocytes entering diplotene on day 18 than on day 16 of gestation. However, Speed and Chandley (1983) were unable to confirm Jagiello and Fang's observation, and several studies of aging female mice and hamsters did not find a correlation between univalent formation at meiosis I and aneusomy later in meiosis or in early embryonic stages (Polani and Jagiello, 1976; Speed, 1977; Sugawara and Mikamo, 1983). Thus, the validity of the model, as well as the contribution of chiasma loss to age-dependent trisomy, remains unproven.

Very few data are available from humans on the possible relationship between chiasma frequency and nondisjunction. Based on data from spontaneous abortions, Hassold *et al.* (1980) suggested that heterogeneous maternal age effects among autosomal trisomies could reflect variation in chiasma frequency among chromosomes. If maternal age-related nondisjunction ensued from loss of chiasmata with age, the effect should be most pronounced among the smallest chromsomes with the fewest chiasmata. Indeed, an inverse correlation exists between the estimated number of chiasmata for a particular chromosome (Laurie and Hulten, 1985) and the mean maternal age of trisomy for that chromosome [for review, see Hassold (1986)].

In a study of 34 families, Antonarakis and co-workers suggested that recombination is depressed on the chromosome 21 involved in nondisjunction (Antonarakis *et al.*, 1986; Warren *et al.*, 1987). In addition to small sample size, there were two major technical limitations to their study. First, they used markers that did not span the terminal third of 21q. Since the linkage map of chromosome 21 (Tanzi *et al.*, submitted) shows a high frequency of terminal chiasmata on 21q, this issue must be addressed using probes spanning the length of 21q. Second, pericentromeric markers were not used to determine the meiotic stage of nondisjunction, an essential feature for this type of analysis. In their report, the 21q sequence CW21pc was used as a pericentromeric marker. CW21pc was linked to the proximal 21q marker D21S13 at a distance of 14 cM (Warren *et al.*, 1987). Warren *et al.* (1987) favored the relative order cen-CW21pc-(D21S1/D21S11) over cen-D21S13-D21S1/D21S11-CW21pc, and therefore used CW21pc as a pericentromeric marker. However, the number of informative meioses was small (Warren *et al.*, 1987), so that the ratio favoring this order was only 1.5/1 in three-point crosses and 2/1 in four-point crosses. In contrast, unpublished data of R. E. Tanzi (personal communication) with a larger number of informative events demonstrates that the CW21pc is ~15 cM distal to 21-4U/D21S13. Thus, the order of markers on 21q is: cen-(21-4U/D21S13)-15 cM-CW21pc, placing CW21pc at a substantial distance from the centromere. Based on the distal assignment of CW21pc, a comparison between the linkage map of Tanzi *et al.* with the data of Warren *et al.* (1987) demonstrates that although Warren *et al.* (1987) did observe fewer crossovers on nondisjoined than on control chromosomes 21, the numbers are small and scatter is evident. The magnitude of the increment of crossover frequency in the control values compared to the linkage map is as great as the decrement of crossover frequency in their nondisjoined chromosomes compared to the linkage map of Tanzi *et al.* Since it is unlikely that crossing over is increased in the chromosomes not involved in nondisjunction, this argues that the increment between the control data and the known linkage map must be due to small sample size or to unappreciated biases in the study. If so, then the decrement between the nondisjoined chromosome data is subject to the same criticism of small sample size, consistent with the marginal statistical significance reported by Warren *et al.* (1987). These deficiencies can only be met by studying a larger sample size, by using probes spanning 21q, and by jointly using both 21p chromosome heteromorphisms and 21q DNA polymorphisms tightly linked to the centromere. Our own limited data using both heteromorphisms and DNA polymorphisms on chromosomes X, 13, and 21 (Hassold *et al.*, 1987; Stewart *et al.*, 1988) did not detect an obvious suppression of recombination on nondisjoined chromosomes. In trisomy 13, recombination was detected in three of five cases of meiosis I origin, and on chromosome 21 we have unequivocal evidence of crossovers on nondisjoined chromosomes 21, including a nondisjoined chromosome that resulted from a maternal meiosis I error (see pilot study cited on p. 123).

The Effect of the Parental Origin of Trisomy on the Phenotype of the Conceptus

It is generally assumed, at least for mammals, that the parental origin of a gene does not affect its expression. However, recent evidence from studies of human spontaneous abortions and studies of the mouse have cast doubt on this assumption. For example, we now know that the phenotype associated with spontaneously aborted triploids varies depending on the origin of the extra haploid set. Specifically, paternal triploids typically have an abnormal placenta and are characterized as partial hydatidiform moles, while maternal triploids do not fall into this category (Jacobs *et al.*, 1982). Furthermore, the paternal triploids usually abort later in pregnancy than maternal triploids.

Several observations indicate that murine genes may be expressed differentially, depending on the parental source. First, the experiments using artificially produced diploid androgenomes and genogenomes (i.e., embryos consisting only of two paternal genomes and embryos consisting only of two maternal genomes), it is clear that both types of embryos are inviable (McGrath and Solter, 1984). Therefore, both paternal and maternal genomes are required for normal embryonic development. Second, breeding studies utilizing different translocations have demonstrated chromosome-specific parental origin effects; i.e., the phenotype associated with maternal duplication/paternal deficiency for a specific chromosome region often differs from the reciprocal paternal duplication/maternal deficiency (Cattanach and Kirk, 1985; Searle and Beechey, 1985). Third, recent studies of transgenic mice demonstrate that for certain transgenes, the methylation patterns change in a predictable manner, depending on whether the transgene is inherited through the father or the mother (Reik *et al.*, 1987; Sapienza *et al.*, 1987).

These observations provide the rationale for suggesting that the phenotype associated with maternal trisomy 21 could differ from cases of paternal origin. A large-scale study of nondisjunction for chromosome 21 presents a special opportunity to study the methylation patterns of DNA probes all along chromosome 21 on chromosomes whose parental origin will be identified, and thereby determine whether methylation is used to mark genetic elements on chromosome 21. Further, it will be possible to examine whether phenotypic severity correlates with parental origin.

MOLECULAR CYTOGENETIC ORGANIZATION OF CHROMOSOME 21: IMPLICATIONS FOR STUDIES OF NONDISJUNCTION

Organization of DNA Sequences on the Short Arms of the Acrocentric Chromosomes

Several families of repeated DNA sequences are found on the short arms of each of the human acrocentric chromosomes, including ribosomal (A. S. Henderson *et al.*, 1972; Evans *et al.*, 1974), satellite (e.g., alphoid) (Kurnit and Maio, 1974; Gosden *et al.*, 1975; Willard and Waye, 1987; Choo *et al.*, 1988), and 724 DNA sequences (Kurnit *et al.*, 1984, 1986). Highly repeated DNAs are characteristic of higher eukaryotes, and appear to have evolved in the main from unequal mitotic crossover events (for reviews see John and Miklos, 1979; Kurnit, 1979). Because intrachromosomal crossovers appear to be more frequent than interchromosomal exchanges, highly repeated DNAs often show chromosomal specificity. Based on this finding, a number of useful probes for the pericentromeric region of individual human chromosomes have been derived by hybridizing alphoid satellite DNA probes from specific chromosomes at high stringency (for review, see Willard and Waye, 1987; Choo *et al.*, 1988).

To date, no single-copy or repeated probes specific for the short arm of chromosome 21 have been isolated. Out of ~70 single-copy, chromosome 21-specific fragments examined, none map to the short arm (Van Keuren *et al.*, 1986; unpublished data of G. Stewart, D. Kurnit, and M. Van Keuren). It is likely that the difficulty in obtaining 21p-specific DNA sequences arises from the increased frequency of mitotic germ-line and meiotic exchanges among the short arms of acrocentric chromosomes. Exchanges between the short arms of human acrocentrics have been documented several times *in vitro* in normal karyotypes (Nielsen *et al.*, 1974; Livingston *et al.*, 1985), and more frequently (as would be expected for mitotic exchanges) in Bloom's syndrome karyotypes (Therman *et al.*, 1981). Indeed, the frequency of these acrocentric exchanges, presumably resulting from nucleolar and/or satellite associations, may preclude the existence of probes unique to the short arm of chromosome 21. Although several low-order repeated DNA sequences have been isolated from 21 p, none map uniquely to 21 p. The most useful 21p probe is D21S5 (Watkins *et al.*, 1985), which hybridizes to a number of *Taq*I restriction fragments on different chromosomes; two of these fragments constitute a restriction fragment length polymorphism (Botstein *et al.*, 1980) that maps to chromosome 21 in a somatic cell mapping panel. Caution is required using the D21S5 polymorphism, as it is not known whether these *Taq*I fragments are represented on other chromosomes in a significant proportion of the population.

At this point, it is unclear whether exchanges among acrocentric chromosomes occur frequently enough to preclude the existence of repeated DNA sequence probes that will be specific for the pericentromeric region of given human acrocentrics. As summarized in a recent review (Willard and Waye, 1987), high-stringency hybridization with chromosome-specific alphoid sequences can be used to obtain polymorphisms for the pericentromeric region of given human chromosomes. Further both alphoid satellite and 724-family DNA sequences manifest distinct patterns in rodent–human hybrid cells carrying individual human acrocentric chromosomes (Jorgensen *et al.*, 1987; Kurnit *et al.*, 1986). Unfortunately, these mapping panels contain only one or a few of each type of acrocentric chromosome, so that it is not possible to discern how universal these preliminary acrocentric-specific patterns are. Indeed, the observation of short-term exchanges among human acrocentric chromosomes in culture makes it unlikely that any acrocentric short-arm configuration will be limited to a single acrocentric in all humans. Nevertheless, within populations or families, it may be feasible to use chromosome 21p polymorphisms detected by alphoid, 724, ribosomal DNA, or other repeated family DNA probes. For example, brilliant fluorescence with distamycin A/DAPI is usually a marker for chromosome 15p (Schweizer *et al.*, 1978; Okamoto *et al.*, 1981), but may be absent on some chromosome 15 short arms (Babu *et al.*, 1986) or present on other acrocentric short arms (Perez-Castillo *et al.*, 1987). However, no such well-characterized 21p DNA polymorphisms are available.

The Interspersed 724 Family on the Acrocentric Short Arms

A HeLa cDNA clone we isolated, pUNC724, detected DNA sequences that comprise a low-order repeated family present in ~10^2 copies per human diploid genome, with multiple copies in the pericentromeric region of each of the human acrocentrics (Kurnit *et al.*, 1984, 1986). From this finding, and from the observation that the family spans over 10^5 base pairs of discrete *Eco*RI fragments, each of which is present in multiple copies on multiple acrocentric chromosomes, the 724 family must span millions of base pairs in the pericentromeric regions of the human acrocentric chromosomes (Kurnit *et al.*, 1984, 1986). This organizational complexity precludes the use of typical 724-family probes to study the segregation of individual acrocentric chromosomes.

The DNA sequences that hybridized with our original clone, pUNC724, comprise a low-order repeated family within the human genome on the short arm of each of the human acrocentrics. To investigate the sequence organization of this family, we utilized a recombination-based assay to retrieve over 100 bacteriophage carrying diverse 724-family members (Kurnit *et al.*, 1984, 1986). Previously, we successfully adapted this recombination-based assay for a number of tasks in human gene mapping, including the retrieval of human DNA sequences from rodent–human libraries (Neve *et al.*, 1983), the determination of copy number of human DNA sequences (Neve and Kurnit, 1983), and chromosome walking (Kurnit *et al.*, 1986).

A 724 probe cloned in the recombination miniplasmid πAN7 (Lutz *et al.*, 1987) was used to screen a genomic human library for phages carrying 724 sequences. DNA from each retrieved phage was digested with *Eco*RI and *Hind*III and subcloned in πAN7. We used the recombination-based assay to eliminate plasmids carrying phage or highly repeated DNA sequences (Neve and Kurnit, 1983). Plasmids devoid of highly repeated human DNA sequences (circles in Fig. 1) were used in turn to screen the genomic library again, and the process was reiterated; the molecular pedigree of our chromosome walking among 724-family members on the short arm of the acrocentrics is shown in Fig. 1 (Kurnit *et al.*, 1986). From this finding, and from the observation that the family spans over 100,000 base pairs of discrete *Eco*RI fragments, each of which is present in multiple copies on multiple acrocentric chromosomes, the 724 family must span millions of base pairs in the pericentromeric regions of the human acrocentric chromosomes. Figure 2 displays the complexity of the *Eco*RI fragments detected by a number of 724-family probes (circled in Fig. 1) isolated during the walking procedure (Kurnit *et al.*, 1986). Based on the somatic cell mapping panel of Van Keuren *et al.* (1986), some of these fragments map distal, whereas others map proximal to the ribosomal locus on 21p. In sum, the 724 family is a family of dispersed repeats spanning the short arms of the human acrocentrics (Kurnit *et al.*, 1984, 1986).

Below, we describe the isolation of distantly related pericentromeric 724-family members that are useful for studies of nondisjunction. By utilizing a chromosome walking (Bender *et al.*, 1983) strategy that relied on recombination *in vivo* to screen a flow-sorted chromosome 21 library with a 724-family probe, we isolated two useful pericentromeric DNA probes on chromosome 21. The flow-sorted chromosome 21 recombinant library was provided by Dr. S. Latt. This library comprises *Hind*III-digested DNA from bivariate, flow-sorted chromosome 21 particles (Lalande *et al.*, 1984) inserted into the *Hind*III cloning vehicle, Charon 21A. Employing a recombination-based assay that can detect as few as 20 homologous base pairs (Watt *et al.*, 1985; Shen and Huang, 1986), we screened for distantly related 724-family members that could not be detected using standard hybridization assays. With a 724 probe in the recombination-based assay, 30 independent phages were retrieved and analyzed. One of these phages (designated phage 21-4) carries a

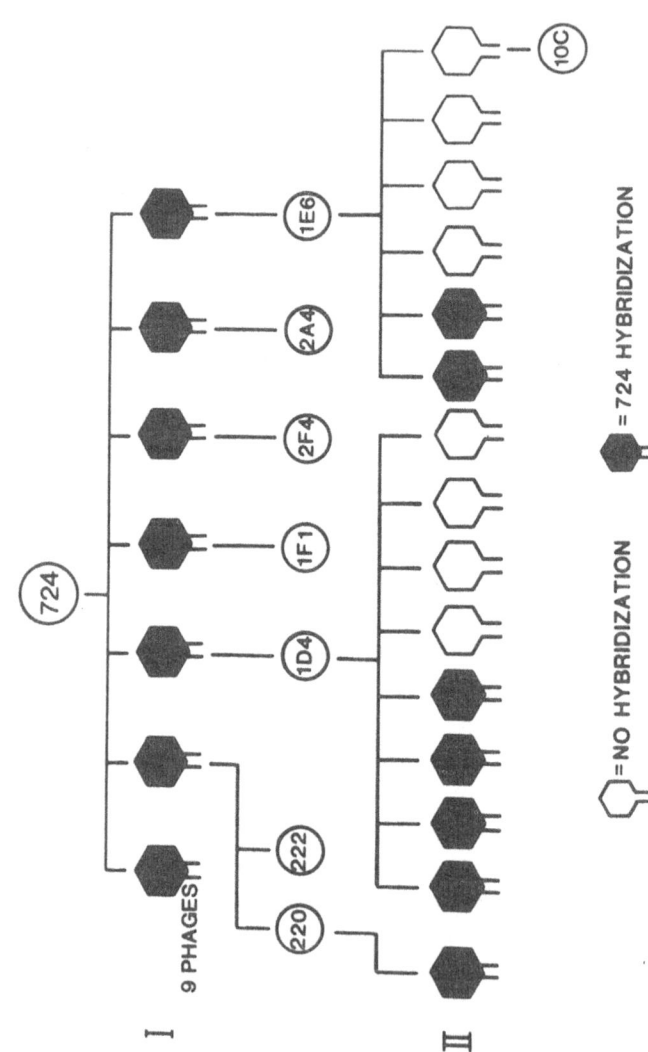

Fig. 1. Molecular pedigree of 724 walking strategy. Circles denote 724-family sequences subcloned in πAN7; hexagons denote recombinant bacteriophages from a human genomic library isolated following homologous recombination with these 724-family sequences. The π724 contains the cDNA fragment subcloned from pUNC724 (Kurnit et al., 1984) into the PstI site of πAN7 (Lutz et al., 1987). The π724 retrieved 50 bacteriophages via recombination from a human genomic library cloned in Charon 4A. Restriction digest analyses of DNA from these phages retrieved by π724 demonstrated that they fell into 15 distinct classes, denoted by the first row of hexagons. DNA from six of these phages was digested with EcoRI and HindIII and subcloned into πAN7. The recombination-based methodology of Neve and Kurnit (1983) was used to distinguish πAN7 plasmids carrying few-copy human DNA inserts. Seven of these are denoted by the next row of circles. The hybridization pattern of each of these radiolabeled miniplasmids to EcoRI digests of human placental DNA is shown in Fig. 2. To walk away from pUNC724-related DNA sequences by isolating phage that no longer shared homology with pUNC724, we hybridized each bacteriophage with radiolabeled pUNC724 cDNA insert subcloned in M13. As expected, all the phages, retrieved in the first round of recombination-based screening hybridized strongly, but several phages in the next rounds of screening did not hybridize with 724. A plasmid carrying single-copy DNA, π10C, was isolated from a phage that showed little cross-reactivity with M13-724, illustrating the interspersion of single-copy DNA sequences adjacent to 724-family members.

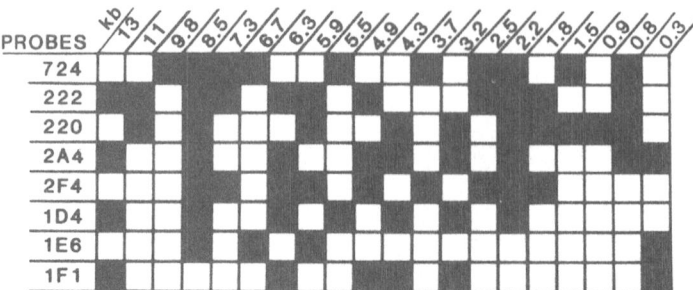

Fig. 2. Hybridization of 724-family members subcloned in πAN7 to EcoRI-digested human DNA. Each of the 724-family members subcloned in πAN7 (depicted as circles in Fig. 1) was radiolabeled and hybridized to EcoRI-digested human placental DNA. The probes are listed in the left-hand column; the size of the EcoRI fragments that comprise the genomic correlates of the 724 family are listed in the top row, with sizes in kilobases. Hybridization to a given EcoRI fragment is denoted by filling in the corresponding box.

DNA fragment (designated p21-4U after subcloning in a plasmid) from chromosome 21q not found on other acrocentric chromosomes. Another phage, designated 21-7, carries a DNA fragment (designated p21-7D after subcloning) that is located in the pericentromeric region of each of the acrocentric chromosomes by *in situ* hybridization. In contrast with p21-4U and 724-family sequences that are homologous to transcribed human and genomic rodent sequences, p21-7D does not hybridize with rodent DNAs under standard hybridization conditions.

Fine structure mapping on chromosome 21 demonstrates the presence of p21-7D sequences on 21p just above the centromere. It appears that the 7D subfamily is present on the long arm as well, so that this subfamily straddles the centromere: p21-7D hybridizes to DNA from a somatic cell hybrid whose sole human complement is a chromosome 21 with a breakpoint on 21q apparently just below the centromere. As expected, there is little or no representation in this hybrid of other 21p DNA sequences, including ribosomal and alphoid DNA families. Due to our inability to ascertain definitively that the human chromosome 21 centromere and all 21p material is absent from this hybrid, we cannot be certain that the 7D family straddles the centromere. Nevertheless, these hybridization data map the 7D subfamily closer to the centromere than other known 21p probes. Although the 7D family is not useful as a chromosome 21-specific probe, it should prove useful in future studies to walk to the centromere of chromosome 21.

The fragment p21-4U is a useful polymorphic probe for the pericentromeric region of chromosome 21. Hybridization of radiolabeled p21-4U to *Eco*RI-digested human genomic DNA labeled a single band at 5 kb that localized uniquely to 21q11 just below the centromere. Mapping was accomplished using both *in situ* hybridization and a somatic cell hybrid panel that dissects chromosome 21 into specific subregions (Van Keuren *et al.*, 1986). Both methods localized p21-4U on the long arm of chromosome 21, just below the centromere in band 21q11. When the enzyme *Msp*I is used to digest human genomic DNA, p21-4U detects a DNA polymorphism, with the less common allele present in ~25% of the Caucasian population. The polymorphism data confirm that p21-4U is a single-copy probe.

We used the *Msp*I polymorphism to place p21-4U on the linkage map of chromosome 21 (Tanzi *et al.*, submitted). This genetic mapping confirms the assignment of p21-4U to the most proximal portion of the long arm, and confirms the usefulness of another probe on chromosome 21, D21S13 (Krumlauf *et al.*, 1982), which is the most proximal 21q marker on the linkage map of Tanzi *et al.* (submitted); there were no recombination events between p21-4U and D21S13 in 29 informative meioses (R. Tanzi, personal communication). The lack of significant linkage disequilibrium between the polymorphisms detected by p21-4U and D21S13 enables us to use these probes jointly to establish a highly informative haplotype. With this pericentromeric 21q haplotype, we distinguish chromosome 21 homologues in a significant plurality of subjects.

Figure 3 summarizes the molecular organization of DNA sequences in the pericentromeric region of chromosome 21, with the 724-family members outlined in rectangles. This organization suggests the opportunity ultimately to "walk" to the centromere. A plausible walking strategy is to walk toward the centromere from the long arm (from p21-4U and/or D21S13) and to search for candidate clones in cosmids and/or artificial yeast chromosome vectors that carry both p21-7D sequences and single-copy 21q sequences.

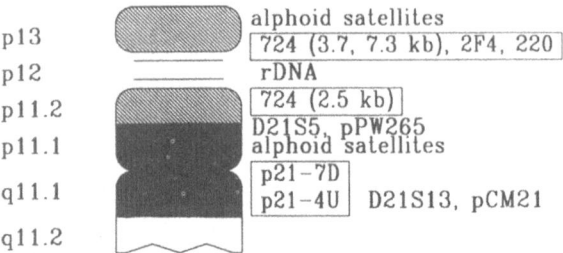

Fig. 3. Molecular organization of the pericentromeric region of human chromosome 21. Subregional localization of DNA probes in the pericentromeric region of chromosome 21 was obtained following hybridization to the somatic cell-mapping panel of Van Keuren *et al.* (1986). Members of the 724 family are outlined in rectangles. The localization of p21-7D and p21-4U was confirmed by *in situ* hybridization (unpublished data of U. Tantravahi); the localization of D21S13 [and its cDNA correlate, pCM21 (Neve *et al.*, 1986)] was based on the finding that p21-4U and D21S13 showed no recombinants from 29 informative meiotic events.

Isolation of a Large Number of Polymorphic Single-Copy DNA Probes That Span the Long Arm of Chromosome 21

The absence of useful 21p polymorphic DNA sequences restricts the availability of 21p polymorphisms to heteromorphic cytogenetic markers. In contrast, single-copy polymorphic DNA sequences are readily isolated from the long arm of chromosome 21, as 21q is not subject to the frequent exchanges among the acrocentrics described for 21p DNA sequences. The strategy to isolate useful markers on 21q is straightforward: (1) Isolate single-copy DNA sequences on chromosome 21, and (2) screen to determine restriction enzymes that detect polymorphisms present frequently enough in the population to be generally useful. Minor allele frequencies of 0.2 or greater are desirable for nondisjunction studies.

To speed the acquisition of single-copy probes on chromosome 21, we merged two efficient technologies: (1) bivariate flow sorting (Langlois *et al.*, 1982; Donlon *et al.*, 1986) of human metaphase chromosomes to isolate chromosome 21-specific DNA and (2) the recombination-based assay to screen for plasmids carrying single-copy, chromosome 21-specific DNA sequences (Neve and Kurnit, 1983). We thereby isolated 30 single-copy DNA probes on chromosome 21 (Tantravahi *et al.*, 1988). First, bivariate flow sorting was used to obtain chromosome preparations highly enriched for chromosome 21. DNA was isolated from these chromosomes, and cloned into the *supF* miniplasmid πAN7 that carries *supF* for use in the recombination-based assay. We detected few-copy DNA sequences by determining the frequency with which each of 400 human, flow-sorted DNA inserts that were subcloned in πAN7 retrieved bacteriophages from a human bacteriophage library: human DNA sequences that recombined infrequently were judged not to be repeated. Seventy-seven of 400 plasmids yielded REP numbers between 1 and 9 (Neve and Kurnit, 1983), and were thereby judged likely to carry few-copy DNA sequences. Rejecting plasmids that carried inserts too short for useful hybridization studies and/or inserts on chromosomes other than chromosome 21, we achieved the rapid isolation of 30 useful single-copy probes on chromosome 21.

These single-copy probes were screened with 40 restriction enzymes to find probe–enzyme combinations that detect useful restriction fragment length polymorphisms. To obtain polymorphisms with useful minor allele frequencies, screening panels were constructed with DNA from five different individuals. The DNA from each is digested with each of the 40 restriction enzymes we utilize, electrophoresed, and transferred to nylon membranes that can be rehybridized at least 20 times (Genatran, Plasco Inc., Woburn, MA). Aldridge *et al.* (1984) demonstrated that such small screening panels can detect over 90% of useful probe–enzyme combinations. Once a potentially useful polymorphism is detected on the screening panel, the frequency of the polymorphism is determined on larger panels of 30 unrelated subjects digested with that particular enzyme. In this fashion, we screened our 30 single-copy probes and obtained useful polymorphisms with 15 of these probes. Coupled with the multiple existing polymorphic markers made available to us from other laboratories (P. Watkins, R. Tanzi, J. Gusella, Y. Groner, T. Springer, J. Piatigorsky, P. Takis, S. Antonarakis, and D. Cox), we have over 60 polymorphic markers on chromosome 21, which have been subregionally mapped using linkage, *in situ* hybridization, and/or somatic cell mapping. The localization of some of these polymorphic 21q DNA markers is summarized in Fig. 4.

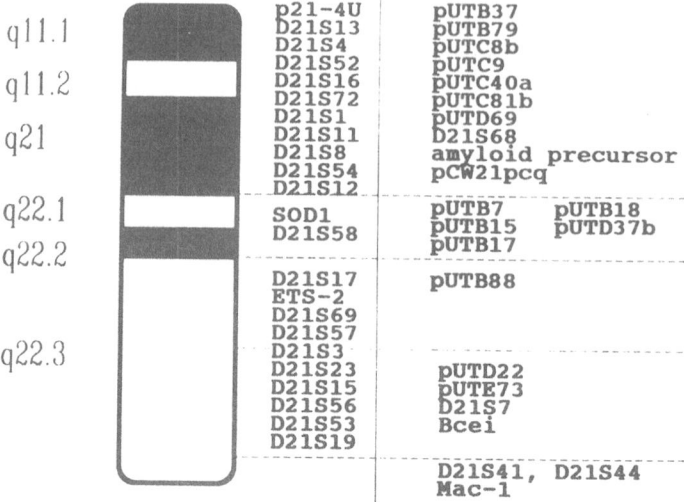

Fig. 4.   Polymorphic probes on chromosome 21. This figure summarizes polymorphic single-copy DNA probes on chromosome 21 currently available for nondisjunction studies. All probes have been mapped into one of five subregions on the long arm of chromosome 21 using the somatic cell panel of Van Keuren *et al.* (1986) plus one additional somatic cell hybrid with a breakpoint in the distal portion of 21q22.3. Probes in the left-hand column have been ordered on the linkage map of Tanzi *et al.* (submitted). Probes in the right-hand column have not yet been ordered by linkage, so that their order within a subregion is not yet defined. The salient point is that sufficient subregionally mapped polymorphic DNA probes spanning the long arm of chromosome 21 are now available for molecular studies of nondisjunction. This list includes probes provided by P. Watkins, R. Tanzi, J. Gusella, Y. Groner, T. Springer, T. Papas, S. Antonarakis, D. Cox, P. Chambon, and U. Tantravahi.

We note that four different questions are to be addressed with DNA polymorphisms, each of which requires somewhat different groupings of DNA probes.

1. The parental origin of nondisjunction. This question may be answered with any single-copy DNA probe on chromosome 21, and is the most demanding in terms of the allelic patterns in mother, father, and child required to be informative. Here the goal is to utilize as many markers as feasible. Fortunately, an adequate number of well-characterized, subregionally mapped, chromosome 21-specific, polymorphic markers is now available (Fig. 4). Given the number of markers available, the efficiency of determining the parental origin of nondisjunction will approach 100%.

2. The meiotic stage during which nondisjunction occurs. Markers for the pericentromeric region are essential to determine how nondisjunction originated at the centromere in each family. To perform these studies adequately, it is necessary to sandwich the centromere between closely linked markers on both the short and long arms, allowing the detection of crossover events between the centromere and either of the markers. This is now feasible using cytogenetic heteromorphisms on one hand and proximal 21q DNA polymorphisms on the other. In particular, the p21-4U/D21S13 is an excellent pericentromeric 21q haplotype, which we will expand in the near future to obtain more polymorphisms closer to the centromere with the goal of making most families informative for at least one pericentromeric locus in 21q11.

The absence of single-copy probes unique to the short arm of chromosome 21 (Van Keuren *et al.*, 1986; Watkins *et al.*, 1985; Human Gene Mapping 8, 1985) requires cytogenetic heteromorphisms to mark the short arm of chromosome 21 in nondisjunction studies. Heteromorphisms are obtained most efficiently by using both Q-banding (Caspersson *et al.*, 1970) and NOR-banding (Howell *et al.*, 1975) on the same slide. The current approach is therefore joint use of careful cytogenetics, done by multiple observers with both Q-bands and silver staining, coupled with analysis of multiple DNA polymorphisms, including the p21-4U/D21S13 haplotype. Only by the simultaneous use of flanking markers on 21p (cytogenetic heteromorphisms) and 21q11 (DNA markers) can the question of meiotic stage be addressed to eliminate confounding effects due to crossovers between the centromere and the polymorphic markers.

3. Recombination during nondisjunction. Answering this question requires polymorphic markers that span the length of chromosome 21. In particular, given the high frequency of terminal chiasmata that exists on the chromosome 21 linkage map, probes at the telomeric end of the 21q linkage map are desired. Probes in the telomeric region of 21q are identified by hybridizing single-copy 21q DNA probes to DNA from a hybrid cell line, Raj5BE, whose sole human chromosome 21 is a translocation between chromosomes 21 and 22 (Pinkerton *et al.*, 1984). The Raj5BE hybrid cell line carries all of 21q except the very distal tip, i.e., from the distal portion of 21q22.3 to 21qter (unpublished data of M. Van Keuren). To date, only three 21q DNA probes, D21S44, D21S41, and Mac-1 (the β chain of a leukocyte adhesion moiety (Marlin *et al.*, 1986; Kishimoto *et al.*, 1987), did not hybridize to Raj5BE DNA, assigning these probes to the distal tip of 21q (Fig. 4; our unpublished data). Fortunately, Mac-1 detects two frequent restriction fragment length polymorphisms, using the enzymes *Pst*I and *Stu*I, that do not show significant linkage disequilibrium. Twenty of 26 random individuals were heterozygous for at least one of the Mac-1 polymorphisms. Just as p21-4U (*Msp*I) and D21S13 (*Taq*I) comprise a useful paracentomeric haplotype, Mac-1 (*Pst*I) and Mac-1 (*Stu*I) comprise a useful paratelomeric haplotype.

4. Are specific DNA haplotypes associated with nondisjunction? Antonarakis and co-workers have recently suggested that specific DNA polymorphic haplotypes on chromosome 21q are associated with increased risk for nondisjunction of this chromosome (Antonarakis *et al.*, 1985). However, examination of a larger cohort of Northern Italian subjects showed no association of these specific DNA haplotypes with nondisjunction for chromosome 21 (Sacchi *et al.*, 1988). Thus, even if the results obtained by Antonarakis *et al.* (1985) remain valid after examination of larger numbers of subjects in the Greek population they examined, this association will not be valid for all ethnic groups. These difficulties reinforce the need to utilize probes tightly linked to the centromere in future screens for haplotypes that might be associated with nondisjunction. The availability of the p21-4U/D21S13 haplotype and the likelihood of isolating additional pericentromeric probes by walking out from these loci will permit reexamination of this hypothesis using markers tightly linked to the centromere in larger numbers of families. If pericentromeric polymorphisms associated with nondisjunction are found, they could be used to detect couples with a high risk for offspring with Down syndrome.

Lessons from a Pilot Study

To analyze the origin of nondisjunction in five families with trisomy 21 offspring, Stewart *et al.* (1988) used cytogenetic polymorphisms and 16 polymorphic DNA probes spanning the long arm from 21q11 to 21q22.3. Chromosomes from these families were stained using Q-banding and NOR-banding to detect 21p heteromorphisms. Parental origin was determined via cytogenetic criteria in two of five families, and it was determined that the error occurred in meiosis I in either parent in a third family. DNA analyses assigned parental origin in four of five families; taken together, cytogenetic plus molecular analyses determined parental origin in all five families (Fig. 5).

In family 1, the cytogenetic markers were uninformative, but analysis of the SOD1 locus indicated a paternal meiosis II error. Knowledge that the error was paternal made the pericentromeric marker p21-4U informative, as this marker data assigned a paternal error as a meiosis II event. The simplest explanation for this case is nondisjunction at paternal meiosis II, with no evidence for crossing over between 21q11 and the midportion of 21q.

In both families 2 and 3 the cytogenetic results indicated a maternal meiosis I error, and in family 2 the maternal origin was confirmed with the DNA marker D21S58. There was no evidence in either of these cases for recombination between the two nondisjoined chromosomes, but in family 2 there were no polymorphic loci informative for meiotic stage distal to the D21S1/D21S11 locus, about one-third of the way down the long arm. Future studies on these families will focus on recently acquired distal 21q markers to determine whether a recombination event can be detected.

In family 4 (Figs. 5 and 6), both cytogenetic markers on 21p and the D21S16 DNA marker on the proximal part of the long arm were consistent with a maternal I error. However, two more distal 21q DNA markers, D21S8 and D21S17, indicated a maternal II error. Crossing over between two nondisjoined chromosomes can be detected only when the parent of origin is heterozygous for two or more markers. For example, in cases of maternal origin, a single (or odd number of) crossover(s) is inferred if the mother is heterozygous

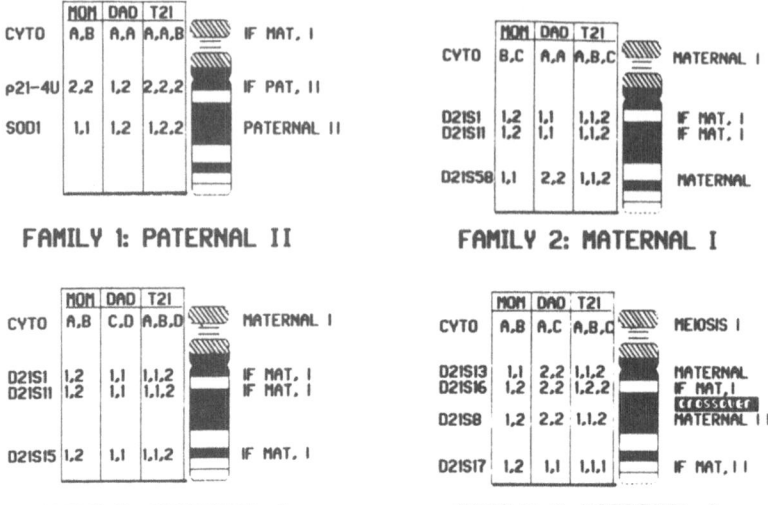

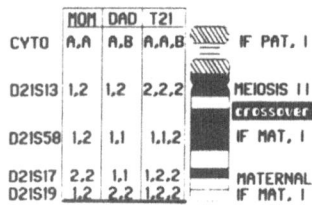

Fig. 5.   Nondisjunction in five Down syndrome families using cytogenetic and DNA polymorphisms. Five families (mother, father, Down syndrome offspring) were studied using cytogenetic heteromorphisms and 16 polymorphic DNA probes spanning chromosome 21 (Stewart *et al.*, 1988). This figure depicts the informative polymorphisms and their relative locations on chromosome 21. In families 4 and 5, crossing over has occurred on a nondisjoined chromosome: in both families, distal probes on 21q are discordant with the stage of meiosis defined by pericentromeric probes.

for two markers, and if the trisomic offspring is homozygous for one marker and heterozygous for the other, having received two maternal chromosomes. Family 4 furnishes an example of such a crossover event: the mother is heterozygous for D21S16 and D21S8, whereas the abortus has both maternal alleles for D21S16 ("maternal I"), but has two copies of a single maternal allele for D21S8 ("ma-

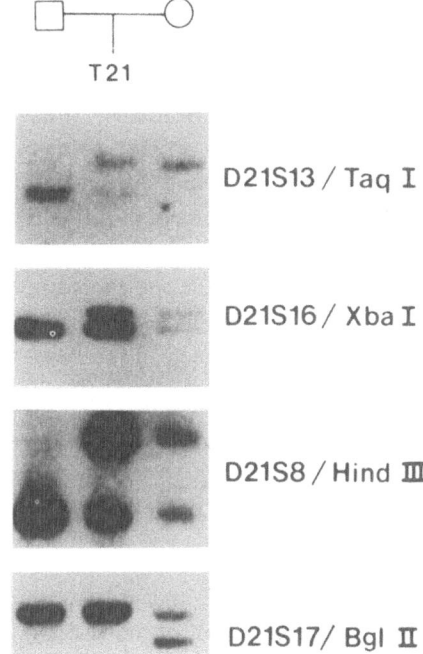

T 21

D21S13 / Taq I

D21S16 / Xba I

D21S8 / Hind Ⅲ

D21S17 / Bgl Ⅱ

Fig. 6. Informative restriction length fragment polymorphisms in family 4 (Fig. 5). The Southern hybridizations for the informative probes in family 4 (see Fig. 5) are shown.

ternal II''). Therefore a crossover must have occurred on a nondisjoined chromosome between the loci identified by D21S16 and D21S8.

In family 5, D21S17 detected a maternal error. In this family, the proximal 21q DNA marker D21S13 indicated a meiosis II error, whereas the more distal 21q markers D21S58 and D21S19 were consistent with an error at maternal meiosis I. The simplest explanation, which invokes a single crossover for this case, is an error at maternal meiosis II and a crossover between the 21q11 marker D21S13 and the mid-long-arm marker D21S58.

These analyses demonstrate the power of combining molecular and cytogenetic studies of nondisjunction. Using a fraction of available DNA probes, it was possible to assign the parental origin of nondisjunction in four of five families, and cytogenetic heteromorphisms defined the last case. In all five families, the meiotic stage was determined using markers tightly linked to the centromere, i.e.,

chromosome heteromorphisms on 21p and/or DNA markers on
21q11. In all informative cases, the molecular analysis using proximal 21q DNA markers were consistent with the cytogenetic analysis
using 21p heteromorphisms. These limited data are consistent with
a low rate of recombination in the pericentromeric area. In turn,
such a low rate would agree with the assertion that meiotic crossovers occur rarely in constitutive heterochromatin (John and Miklos,
1979; Kurnit, 1979). In this small study, there were no contradictions
between cytogenetic and molecular studies. Extension of this pilot
study using more DNA probes on more families will address many
of the questions listed at the beginning of this review.

AN EXPERIMENTAL DESIGN TO ANSWER THE BASIC QUESTIONS RELATED TO NONDISJUNCTION

The projected success of a population-based, molecular and cytogenetic analysis of nondisjunction for chromosome 21 is based on
the advances reviewed above, including:

1. Multiple polymorphic DNA probes that span the long arm
   of chromosome 21.
2. Ordering of these probes via both a somatic cell mapping
   panel (Van Keuren et al., 1986) and a linkage map (Tanzi et
   al., submitted).
3. Informative pericentromeric and paratelomeric polymorphisms.
4. A sequential Q-stain and NOR chromosome-banding technique (Lau et al., 1978) that maximizes the informativeness
   of cytogenetic heteromorphism data on chromosome 21.

We estimate that an adequate study should analyze 500 cases
of Down syndrome. For each case, chromosomes and DNA from
the index Down syndrome child and from both parents should be
studied. A key feature of such a study will be the ability to examine
a large number of families over all maternal age ranges. This will
yield statistically meaningful comparisons, and should yield reason-

able numbers to examine the distribution of errors (maternal I, maternal II, paternal I, paternal II) within different age categories. Only by studying such a large number of subjects with a comprehensive protocol can one answer questions relating to nondisjunction definitely, as well as utilize the database to answer a number of ancillary questions not usually addressed in studies of nondisjunction.

Complete Ascertainment of Parental Origin and Meiotic Stage of Nondisjunction

Complete and accurate assessment of both the parental origin and meiotic stage of nondisjunction is required in order to distinghish between the "older egg" and "relaxed selection" models, to evaluate putative etiological agents, and to assess the role of recombinational errors in nondisjunction. The large number of available polymorphic DNA markers on chromosome 21 is sufficient to achieve the determination of parental origin in virtually all cases (Stewart, 1984; Stewart *et al.*, 1985, 1988). Assume:

1. Hardy–Weinberg equilibrium for a two-allele polymorphic system.
2. Frequency of the two alleles $= p$ and q, respectively.
3. Eighty percent of nondisjunction errors yielding trisomy 21 occur in meiosis I, and 20% of errors occur in meiosis II.

The parental origin of nondisjunction can be ascertained for both meiosis I and meiosis II errors whenever both parents are homozygous for different alleles. The frequency of such matings is $2p^2q^2$.

Further, the parental origin of nondisjunction can be ascertained for meiosis II errors when the error occurs in a heterozygous parent that results in duplication of the allele not found in the other (homozygous) parent. This methodology works for meiosis I errors, but not for meiosis II errors, when a crossover has occurred between the centromere and the probe locus on the relevant chromosome; this case, which would be favorable to our calculation, is neglected in the equations below. The frequency of such informative matings is

$$0.5[p^2(2pq) + q^2(2pq)] = pq(p^2 + q^2)$$

The probability P that a given probe can determine the parental origin is

$$P = 2p^2q^2 + 0.2 [pq(p^2 + q^2)]$$

Using an average minor allele frequency of 0.2 ($q = 0.2$) yields $P = 0.073$/probe. Using up to 50 probes for each family indicates that the probability that parental origin cannot be determined is low, i.e., $(1-0.073)^{50} = \sim1/50$. Further, since cytogenetic heteromorphisms (which determine parental origin in at least 50% of cases) can also be examined, virtually complete ascertainment of parental origin is now feasible. These expectations were confirmed in our pilot study, in which we successfully determined parental origin in all five families examined with cytogenetic heteromorphisms and 16 polymorphic DNA probes (Fig. 5). Such complete ascertainment eliminates biases that underestimate meiosis I errors due to incomplete informativeness (Langenbeck et al., 1976).

The determination of meiotic stage is assisted by a thorough ascertainment of parental origin. Many probes do not by themselves distinguish whether nondisjunction occurred in egg or sperm, but once the source of parental error is known, these probes may reveal the stage of meiosis at which nondisjunction occurs (Fig. 5). In particular, increasing the informativeness for meiotic stage of pericentromeric markers such as p21-4U and D21S13 is especially helpful in sandwiching the centromere between polymorphic markers on 21p and 21q. Virtual certainty for determination of meiotic stage is obtained when long- and short-arm markers close to the centromere are concordant.

The Maternal Age Conundrum: Is the Maternal Age Effect due to Increased Production of Abnormal Eggs or Decreased Destruction of Abnormal Embryos?

The definitive study to resolve this issue will require virtually complete ascertainment of the parental source of trisomy in a large number of Down syndrome subjects. The "older egg" model predicts that the proprotion of maternal meiosis I errors will correlate with the advanced maternal age curve for Down Syndrome births; the "relaxed selection" model predicts no maternal age effect on the proportion of maternal meiosis I errors. A large number of families will be required in order to distinguish between the two models because maternal meiosis I errors comprise a large percentage of all nondisjunction events; as a result, the baseline number of maternal meiosis I errors is high in all groups, making it more difficult to detect an increased frequency of such errors in older mothers; the mathematical correlates of this difficulty have been derived that show how small errors in assignment of meiotic errors (Carothers, 1987) or uniformativeness (Langenbeck et al., 1976) can lead to significant biases. Distinction between the two models must be made to determine whether longer range studies of the maternal age effect should focus on abnormalities of egg production or embryo rejection.

Identification of Couples at High Risk for Trisomy 21 Offspring

Antonarakis and co-workers reported that particular polymorphic haplotypes detected by probes pPW228C (D21S1) and pPW236B (D21S11) were found more frequently in the chromosomes 21 that underwent nondisjunction in Down syndrome subjects than in control chromosomes 21. They speculated that these polymorphisms are associated with an increased risk of having offspring with Down syndrome. Since the study involved small numbers of subjects, and the probes used are distant [at least 15 cM from the centromere (R. Tanzi, personal communication)], this conclusion remains problematic. However, the concept of looking for polymorphisms that are linked tightly to the centromere and that are associated with an increased risk for nondisjunction is sound. The attempt to find haplotypes associated with increased nondisjunction should be pursued in future studies using larger cohorts and haplotypes on 21q closely linked to the centromere. Such studies will be permitted by the availability of the p21-4U/D21S13 haplotype and by the potential to walk from these loci ever closer to the centromere on 21q.

Is There a Correlation between Crossing Over and Nondisjunction on Chromosome 21?

A useful linkage map of DNA markers spanning the long arm of chromosome 21 has been constructed using a collection of approximately 25 polymorphic DNA probes (Tanzi *et al.*, submitted). In addition to these classical linkage studies, nondisjunction studies can serve as a form of centromere mapping, yielding data that can determine linkage among polymorphic DNA markers on 21q. However, for the present review it is more important to note that centromere mapping provides the method for examining the relationship between crossing over and nondisjunction.

The centromere mapping method is essentially the same as that previously described for ovarian teratomas (Ott *et al.*, 1976), with the application to trisomy recently discussed by Morton *et al.* (1985) and Slaugenhaupt and Chakravarti (1986). Briefly, the method depends on the fact that two of the four products of meiosis are present in the trisomic offspring; by analogy with tetrad analysis in fungi, the two nondisjoined chromosomes represent an unordered half-tetrad. In this situation, information on centromere–gene distances can be obtained if the parent and meiotic stage of origin of nondisjunction for chromosome 21 are known. A nondisjunction study on chromosome 21 is ideally designed for this purpose, given the ability to span chromosome 21q with a reasonable number of ordered probes that detect polymorphisms (Fig. 4). After assigning the meiotic stage using pericentromeric markers, one searches for more distal markers that are discordant for meiotic stage with the pericentromeric markers; this is illustrated in family 4, where pericentromeric markers indicated a meiosis I error, whereas the more distal probes specified meiosis II. Knowing the order of the probes on chromosome 21, one could localize a crossover event between D21S16 and D21S8 in family 4 (Fig. 5).

Centromeric distances are determined by evaluating the level of heterozygosity among trisomic polymorphisms for which the parent of origin is known to be heterozygous. In centromere mapping, the specific variable being estimated is y, which is a measure of the probability that heterozygosity in the nondisjoining parent is reduced to homozygosity in the disomic gamete. For nondisjunction at meiosis II, the frequency of nonreduction is equal to y and for meiosis I errors the frequency of nonreduction is equal to $1-y/2$ (Shahar and Morton, 1986). Recently, Shahar and Morton (1986) generalized the formulas of Jacobs and Morton (1977) on the origin of trisomy, providing a mechanism for considering recombination between the centromere and a marker locus. Thus, for a given locus, information on y can be converted into lod scores for recombination with the centromere, i.e.,

$$Z(y) = \log_{10} [L(y)/L(2/3)]$$

where $y = 2/3$ represents lack of linkage between the centromere and the marker, and $L(y)$ is the likelihood function for all cases studied.

The possible association between errors in pairing or crossing over and nondisjunction can be evaluated by comparing centromere mapping data of trisomies originating at meiosis I with appropriate controls. Shahar and Morton (1986) have shown that for map distances up to 30 cM the approximation $y = 2\theta$ holds. Thus, over short distances conventional linkage data on chromosome 21 can be compared to linkage data generated by chromosome mapping. Further, centromere mapping data derived from studies of trisomies of meiosis I origin can be compared with two different types of centromere mapping control data, namely triploids of meiosis I and II origin and trisomies of meiosis II origin. If failure to pair or exchange is an important contributor to meiosis I, it should be possible to demonstrate a significant effect with a very small number of controls of this type.

The Effect of Parental Origin of Trisomy on the Phenotype of the Conceptus

It has been observed using both murine models of aneusomy and transgenic mice that differential activity of parts of the autosomal genome may be influenced by the parental origin of the material (Cattanach and Kirk, 1985; Searle and Beechey, 1985). Therefore, it is conceivable that the effects of chromosomal imbalance may be influenced by which parent contributes the aneusomic material. A nondisjunction study can address this issue in several ways. Phenotypic severity can be correlated with the parental origin of the extra chromosome 21 by determining whether the phenotype of trisomy 21 has significantly different manifestations depending on whether mother or father is the source of the aneusomic chromosome 21. Another way of asking whether the parental soure of nondisjunction affects outcome is to use viability through fetal life as a marker for outcome: after matching the groups for maternal age at conception, the frequency of maternal errors is compared in liveborn subjects with Down syndrome and in trisomy 21 abortuses. Hybridization to chromosome 21-specific DNA probes with both *Hpa*II (methylation-sensitive) and *Msp*I (methylation-insensitive) isoschizomers (Waalwijk and Flavell, 1978) can be compared to determine broad patterns of methylation on chromosome 21. In this manner, one can search for differential methylation of subregions of chromosome 21 in sperm and eggs. In at least one case of failure of a maternally inherited transgene to express when a paternally inherited transgene does express, differential methylation patterns in sperm and egg were concordant with expression patterns (Reik *et al.*, 1987; Sapienza *et al.*, 1987). Using dosage and the knowledge of which parent contributes the extra chromosome, one can determine whether methylation patterns are different on chromosomes 21 inherited from mother and father. The ability to examine this question for human autosomes is permitted by the unique set of circumstances where knowledge of both dosage and parental origin of an extra autosome is available. Employment of each of the above strategies in a large-scale study of nondisjunction for chromosome 21 could detect evidence for parental imprinting in man.

OVERVIEW

The time is now ripe to combine molecular and cytogenetic approaches to ask and answer fundamental questions relating to nondisjunction. To date, much has been alleged and little proven. While it is clear that nondisjunction for chromosome 21 involves a significant fraction of paternal errors (20%), other basic questions remain unresolved. The two major outstanding questions are: (1) Is the maternal age effect due to abnormalities of oogenesis in older mothers or to relaxed selection in older mothers, and (2) is recombination altered globally or in a subregion of chromosome 21? The unique confluence of materiel and approaches required to answer these fundamental questions now exists. Recent advances in our understanding of the molecular organization of chromosome 21 have yielded the requisite collection of ordered polymorphic DNA probes on chromosome 21, including useful pericentromeric and paratelomeric haplotypes. The answers to several outstanding questions relating to nondisjunction of chromosome 21 are at hand.

ACKNOWLEDGMENTS.   Research support was provided through NIH R01 HD20118, R01 HL 37703, and HD21341 and March of Dimes Clinical Research G6-501. D. M. K. is an Investigator, and G. D. S. is an Associate, Howard Hughes Medical Institute.

REFERENCES

Aldridge, J., Kunkel, L., Bruns, G., Tantravahi, U., Lalande, M., Brewster, T., Moreau, E., Wilson, M., Bromley, W., Latt, S. A., and Lange, K., 1984, A strategy to reveal high frequency restriction fragment length polymorphisms along the human X chromosome, *Am. J. Hum. Genet.* **376**:546–564.

Alfi, O. S., Chang, R., and Azen, S. P., 1980, Evidence for genetic control of nondisjunction in man, *Am. J. Hum. Genet.* **32**:477–483.

Antonarakis, S. E., Kittur, S. D., Metaxotou, C., Watkins, P. C., and Patel, A. S., 1985, Analysis of DNA haplotypes suggests a genetic predisposition to trisomy 21 associated with DNA sequences on chromosome 21, *Proc. Natl. Acad. Sci. USA* **82**:3360–3364.

Antonarakis, S. E., Chakravarti, A., Warren, A. C., Slaugenhaupt, S. A., Wong, C., Halloran, S. L., and Metaxotou, C., 1986, Reduced recombination rate on chromosomes 21 that have undergone nondisjunction, *Cold Spring Harbor Symp. Quant. Biol.* **51**:185–190.

Ayme, S., and Lippman-Hand, A., 1982, Maternal-age effect in aneuploidy: Does altered embryonic selection play a role? *Am. J. Hum. Genet.* **34**:558–565.

Ayme, S., Baccichetti, C., Bricarelli, F. D., Dallapiccola, B., Lungarotti, D., Mikkelsen, M., and Nevin, M., 1986, Factors involved in chromosomal nondisjunction: A European collaborative study, in: *EEC 7th International Congress of Human Genetics, Abstracts*, Part I:C IV.19.

Babu, A., Macera, M. J., and Verma, R. S., 1986, Intensity heteromorphisms of human chromosome 15p by DA/DAPI technique, *Hum. Genet.* **73**:298–300.

Bender, W., Akam, M., Karch, F., Beachy, P. A., Peifer, M., and Spierer, P., 1983, Molecular genetics of the bithorax complex in *Drosophila melanogaster, Science* **221**:23–29.

Biddle, F., Eates, B., and Oland, L., 1986, Strain difference in survival of XO embryos in the mouse, *Am. J. Hum. Genet.* **39**:A104.

Botstein, D., White, R. L., Skolnick, M., and Davis, R. W., 1980, Construction of a genetic linkage map in man using restriction fragment length polymorphisms, *Am. J. Hum. Genet.* **32**:314–331.

Bott, C. E., Sekhon, B. S., and Lubs, H. A., 1975, Unexpected high frequency of paternal origin of trisomy 21, *Am. J. Hum. Genet.* **27**:20A.

Boué, J. G., and Boué, A., 1973, Increased frequency of chromosomal anomalies after induced ovulation, *Lancet* i:679–680.

Boué, J., Boué, A., and Lazar, P., 1975, Retrospective and prospective epidemiological studies of 1,506 karyotyped spontaneous abortions, *Teratology* **12**:11–26.

Bridges, C. B., 1916, Nondisjunction as proof of the chromosome theory of heredity, *Genetics* **1**:1–52, 107–163.

Carr, D. H., and Gedeon, M. M., 1978, Q-banding of chromosomes in human spontaneous abortions, *Can. J. Genet. Cytol.* **20**:415–425.

Carothers, A., 1987, Down syndrome and maternal age: The effect of erroneous assignment of parental origin, *Am. J. Hum. Genet.* **40**:147–150.

Caspersson, T., Zech, L., Johansson, C., and Modest, E. J., 1970, Identification of human chromosomes by DNA-binding fluorescent agents, *Chromosoma* **30**:215–227.

Cattanach, B. M., and Kirk, M., 1985, Differential activity of maternally and paternally derived chromosome regions in mice, *Nature* **315**:496–498.

Choo, K. H., Vissel, B., Brown, R., Filby, R. G., and Earle, E., 1988, Homologous alpha satellite sequences on human acrocentric chromosomes with selectivity of chromosomes 13, 14 and 21: Implications for recombination between nonhomologues and Robertsonian translocations, *Nucleic Acids Res.* **16**:1273–1284.

Cuckle, H. S., Wald, N. J., and Lindenbaum, R. H., 1984, Maternal serum alphafetoprotein measurement: A screening test for Down syndrome, *Lancet* i:926–929.

Del Mazo, J., Castillo, A. M., and Abrisqueta, J. A., 1982, Trisomy 21: Origin of nondisjunction, *Hum. Genet.* **63**:316–320.

DiMaio, M. S., Baumgarten, A., Greenstein, R. M., Saal, H. M., and Mahoney, M. J., 1987, Screening for fetal Down's syndrome in pregnancy by measuring maternal serum alpha-fetoprotein levels, *N. Engl. J. Med.* **317**:342–346.

Donlon, T. A., Lalande, M., Wyman, A., Bruns, G., and Latt, S. A., 1986, Isolation of molecular probes associated with the chromosome #15 instability in the Prader–Willi syndrome, *Proc. Natl. Acad. Sci. USA* **83**:4409–4412.

Erickson, J. D., 1981, Paternal age and Down syndrome, *Am. J. Hum. Genet.* **31**:489–497.

Evans, H. J., Buckland, R. A., and Pardue, M. L., 1974, Location of the genes coding for 18S and 28S ribosomal RNA in the human genome, *Chromosoma* **48**:405–426.

Ferguson-Smith, M. A., and Handmaker, S. D., 1986, Observations on the satellited human chromosomes, *Lancet* **i**:638.

Flannery, D. B., and Jackson-Cook, C. K., 1986, Thyroid antibodies are an independent risk factor for nondisjunction of chromosome 21, *Am. J. Hum. Genet* **39**(Suppl.):A113.

Ford, J. H., and Lester, P., 1978, Chromosomal variants on nondisjunction, *Cytogenet. Cell Genet.* **21**:300–303.

Gosden, J. R., Mitchell, A. R., Buckland, R. A., Clayton, R. P., and Evan, H. J., 1975, The location of four human satellite DNAs on human chromosomes, *Exp. Cell Res.* **92**:148–158.

Grell, R. F., 1979, Origin of meiotic nondisjunction in *Drosophila* females, *Environ. Health Perspect.* **31**:33–39.

Hamerton, J. L., 1971, *Human Cytogenetics*, Vol. II, *Clinical Cytogenetics*, Academic Press, New York.

Hansson, A., and Mikkelsen, M., 1978, The origin of the extra chromosome 21 in Down syndrome. Studies of fluorescent variants and satellite association in 26 informative families, *Cytogenet. Cell Genet.* **20**:194–203.

Harlap, S., Shiono, P. H., Pellegrin, F., Golbus, M., Bachman, R., Mann, J., Schmidt, L., and Lewis, J. P., 1979, Chromosome abnormalities in oral contraceptive breakthrough pregnancies, *Lancet* **i**:1342–1343.

Hassold, T., 1986, Chromosome abnormalities in human reproductive wastage, *Trends Genet.* **2**:105–110.

Hassold, T. J., Matsuyama, A., Newlands, I. M., Matsuura, J. S., Jacobs, P. A., Manuel, B., and Tsuei, J. A., 1978, Cytogenetic study of spontaneous abortions in Hawaii, *Ann. Hum. Genet.* **41**:443–454.

Hassold, T., Jacobs, P. A., Kline, J., Stein, Z., and Warburton, D., 1980, Effect of maternal age on autosomal trisomies, *Ann. Hum. Genet.* **44**:19–36.

Hassold, T., Jacobs, P. A., and Pettay, D., 1987, Analysis of nucleolar organizing regions in patients of trisomic spontaneous abortions, *Hum. Genet.* **76**:381–384.

Henderson, A. S., Warburton, D., and Atwood, K. C., 1972, Location of ribosomal DNA in the human chromosome complement, *Proc. Natl. Acad. Sci. USA* **69**:3394–3398.

Henderson, S. A., and Edwards, R. G., 1968, Chiasma frequency and maternal age in mammals, *Nature* **218**:22–28.

Hook, E. B., and Regal, R. R., 1984, A search for a paternal-age effect upon cases of 47, + 21 in which the extra chromosome is of paternal origin, *Am. J. Hum. Genet.* **36**:413–421.

Hook, E. B., Cross, P. K., Lamson, S. H., Regal, R. R., Baird, P. A., and Uh, S. H., 1981, Paternal age and Down syndrome in British Columbia, *Am. J. Hum. Genet.* **33**:123–128.

Houghton, J. A., 1981, The study of chromosome nondisjunction in man, *Irish J. Med. Sci.* **150**:357–366.

Howell, W. M., Denton, T. E., and Diamond, J. R., 1975, Differential staining of the satellite regions of human acrocentric chromosomes, *Experientia* **31**:260–262.

Human Gene Mapping 8, 1985, Eighth International Workshop on Human Gene Mapping, *Cytogenetic. Cell Genet.* Vol. 40, Nos. 1–4.

Jackson-Cook, C. K., Flannery, D. B., Corey, L. A., Nance, W. E., and Brown, J. A., 1985, Nucleolar organizer region variants as a risk factor for Down syndrome, *Am. J. Hum. Genet.* **37**:1049–1061.

Jacobs, P. A., and Mayer, M., 1981, The origin of human trisomy: A study of heteromorphisms and satellite associations, *Ann. Hum. Genet.* **45**:49–57.

Jacobs, P. A., and Morton, N. E., 1977, Origin of human trisomies and polyploids, *Hum. Hered.* **27**:59–72.

Jacobs, P. A., Szulman, A. E., Funkhouser, J., Matsuura, J., and Wilson, M. A., 1982, Human triploidy: Relationship between parental origin of the additional haploid complement and development of partial hydatidiform mole, *Ann. Hum. Genet.* **46**:223–232.

Jagiello, G., and Fang, J. S., 1979, Analyses of diplotene chiasma frequencies in mouse ooctyes and spermatocytes in relation to aging and sexual dimorphism, *Cytogenet. Cell Genet.* **23**:53–60.

John, B., and Miklos, G. L. G., 1979, Functional aspects of satellite DNA and heterochromatin, *Int. Rev. Cytol.* **58**:1–114.

Jorgensen, A. L., Jones, C., Bostock, C. J., and Bak, A. L., 1987, Different subfamilies of alphoid repetitive DNA are present on the human and chimpanzee homologous chromosomes 21 and 22, *EMBO J.* **6**:1691–1696.

Juberg, R. C., and Mowrey, P. N., 1983, Origin of nondisjunction in trisomy 21 syndrome. All studies compiled, parental age analysis, and external comparisons, *Am. J. Med. Genet.* **16**:111–116.

Kaufman, M., 1983, Ethanol-induced chromosomal abnormalities at conception, *Nature* **302**:258–260.

Kikuchi, Y., Oishi, H., Tonomura, A., Yamda, K., Tanaka, Y., Kurita, T., and Matsunaga, E., 1969, Translocation Down's syndrome in Japan: Its frequency, mutation rate of translocation and parental age, *Jpn. J. Hum. Genet.* **14**:93–106.

Kishimoto, T. K., O'Connor, K., Lee, A., Roberts, T. M., and Springer, T. A., 1987, Cloning of the β subunit of the leukocyte adhesion proteins: Homology to an extracellular matrix receptor defines a novel supergene family, *Cell* **48**:681–690.

Kline, J., Levin, B., Shrout, P., Stein, Z., Susser, M., and Warburton, D., 1983, Maternal smoking and trisomy among spontaneously aborted conceptions, *Am. J. Hum. Genet.* **35**:421–431.

Krumlauf, R., Jeanpierre, M., and Young, B. D., 1982, Construction and characterization of genomic libraries from specific human chromosomes, *Proc. Natl. Acad. Sci USA* **79**:2971–2975.

Kurnit, D. M., 1979, Satellite DNA and heterochromatin variants: The case for unequal mitotic crossing over, *Hum. Genet.* **47**:169–186.

Kurnit, D. M., and Maio, J. J., 1974, Variable satellite DNA's in the African green monkey, *Cercopithecus aethiops, Chromosoma* **45**:387–400.

Kurnit, D. M., Neve, R. L., Morton, C. C., Bruns, G. A. P., Ma, N. S. F., Cox, D. R., and Klinger, H. P., 1984, Recent evolution of DNA sequence homology in the pericentromeric region of human acrocentric chromosomes, *Cytogenet. Cell Genet.* **38**:99–105.

Kurnit, D. M., Roy, S., Stewart, G. D., Schwedock, J., Neve, R. L., Bruns, G. A. P., Van Keuren, M. L., and Patterson, D., 1986, The 724 family of DNA sequences is interspersed about the pericentromeric regions of human acrocentric chromosomes, *Cytogenet. Cell Genet.* **43**:109–116.

Lalande, M., Dryja, T. P., Schreck, R. R., Shipley, J., Flint, A., and Latt, S. A., 1984, Isolation of human chromosome 13-specific DNA sequences cloned from flow-sorted chromosomes and potentially linked to the retinoblastoma locus, *Cancer Genet. Cytogenet.* **13**:283–296.

Langenbeck, U., Hansmann, I., Hinney, B., and Honig, V., 1976, On the origin of the supernumerary chromosome in autosomal trisomies—With special reference to Down syndrome. A bias in tracing nondisjunction by chromosomal and biochemical polymorphisms, *Hum. Genet.* **33**:89–102.

Langlois, R. G., Yu, L. C., Gray, J. W., and Carrano, A. V., 1982, Quantitative karyotyping of human chromosomes by dual beam flow cytometry, *Proc. Natl. Acad. Sci. USA* **79**:7876–7880.

Lau, Y.-F., Pfeiffer, R. A., Arrighi, F. E., and Hsu, T. C., 1978, Combination of silver and fluorescent staining for metaphase chromosomes, *Am. J. Hum. Genet.* **30**:76–79.

Laurie, D. A., and Hulten, M. A., 1985, Further studies on bivalent chiasma frequency in human males with normal karyotypes, *Ann. Hum. Genet.* **49**:189–201.

Livingston, G. K., Lockey, J. E., Witt, K. S., and Rogers, S. W., 1985, An unstable giant satellite associated with chromosomes 21 and 22 in the same individual, *Am. J. Hum. Genet.* **37**:553–560.

Luthardt, F. W., 1977, Cytogenetic analyses of human oocytes, *Am. J. Hum. Genet.* **29**:71A.

Luthardt, F. W., Palmer, C. G., and Yu, P.-L., 1973, Chiasma and univalent frequencies in aging female mice, *Cytogenet. Cell Genet.* **12**:68–79.

Lutz, C. T., Hollifield, W. C., Seed, B., Davie, J. M., and Huang, H. V., 1987, Syrinx 2A: An improved λ vector designed for screening DNA libraries by recombination *in vivo*, *Proc. Natl. Acad. Sci. USA* **84**:4379–4383.

Magenis, R. E., Overton, K. M., Chamberlin, J., Brady, T., and Lovrien, E., 1977, Prenatal origin of the extra chromosome in Down's syndrome, *Hum. Genet.* **37**:7–16.

Marlin, S. D., Morton, C. C., Anderson, D. C., and Springer, T. A., 1986, LFA-1 immunodeficiency disease. Definition of the genetic defect and chromosomal mapping of a and b subunits of the lymphocyte function-associated antigen 1 (LFA-1) by complementation in hybrid cells, *J. Exp. Med* **164**:855–867.

Mattei, J. F., Ayme, S., Mattei, M. G., and Giraud, F., 1980, Maternal age and origin of nondisjunction in trisomy 21, *J. Med. Genet.* **17**:368–372.

McGrath, J., and Solter, D., 1984, Completion of mouse embryogenesis requires both the maternal and parental genomes, *Cell* **37**:179–183.

Merriam, J. R., and Frost, J. N., 1964, Exchange and nondisjunction of the X-chromosomes in female *Drosophila melanogaster, Genetics* **49**:109–122.

Mikkelsen, M., Hanne, P., Jorgen, G., and Aksel, L., 1980, Nondisjunction in trisomy 21: Study of chromosomal heteromorphisms in 110 families, *Ann. Hum. Genet. Lond.* **4**:17–28.

Morton, N. E., MacLean, C., and Lew, R., 1985, Tests of hypotheses on recombination frequencies, *Genet. Res.* **45**:279–286.

Mottironi, V. D., Hook, E. B., Willey, A. M., Porter, I. H., Swift, R. V., and Hatcher, N. H., 1983, Decreased HLA heterogeneity in parents of children with Down syndrome, *Am. J. Hum. Genet.* **35**:1289–1296.

Neve, R. L., and Kurnit, D. M., 1983, Comparison of sequence repetitiveness of human cDNA and genomic DNA using the recombination miniplasmid, piVX, *Gene* **23**:355–367.

Neve, R. L., Bruns, G. A. P., Dryja, T. P., and Kurnit, D. M., 1983, Retrieval of human DNA from rodent–human libraries by a recombination process, *Gene* **23**:343–354.

Neve, R. L., Stewart, G. D., Newcomb, P., Van Keuren, M. L., Patterson, D., Drabkin, H. A., and Kurnit, D. M., 1986, Human chromosome 21–encoded cDNA clones, *Gene* **49**:361–369.

Nielsen, J., Freidrich, U., Hreidarsson, A. B., Noel, B., Quack, B., and Mottet, J., 1974, Brilliantly fluorescing enlarged short arms D or G, *Lancet* **1**:1049–1050.

Okamoto, E., Miller, D. A., Erlanger, B. F., and Miller, O. J., 1981, Polymorphism of 5-methylcytosine-rich DNA in human acrocentric chromosomes, *Hum. Genet.* **48**:255–259.

Ott, J., Linder, D., McCaw, B. K., Lovrien, E., and Hecht, F., 1976, Estimating distances from the centromere by means of benign ovarian teratomas in man, *Ann. Hum. Genet.* **40**:191–196.

Park, S. C., Mathews, R. A., Zuberbuhler, J. R., Rowe, R. D., Neches, W. H., and Lenox, C. C., 1977, Down syndrome with congenital heart malformation, *Am. J. Dis. Child.* **131**:29–33.

Penrose, L. S., 1933, The relative effect of paternal age and maternal age in mongolism, *J. Genet.* **27**:219–224.

Perez-Castillo, A., Martin-Lucas, M. A., and Abrisqueta, J. A., 1986, New insights into the effects of extra nucleolus organizer regions, *Hum. Genet.* **72**:80–82.

Pinkerton, P. H., London, B., and Senn, J. S., 1984, Chronic myeloid leukemia with a Philadelphia chromosome involving a t(21;22), *Cancer Genet. Cytogenet.* **12**:175–178.

Polani, P. E., and Jagiello, G. M., 1976, Chiasmata, meiotic univalents and age in relationship to aneuploid imbalance in mice, *Cytogenet. Cell Genet.* **16**:505–529.

Pueschel, S. M., 1987, Maternal alpha-fetoprotein screening for Down's syndrome, *N. Engl. J. Med.* **317**:376–378.

Reik, W., Collick, A., Norris, M. L., Barton, S. C., and Surani, M. A., 1987, Genomic imprinting determines methylation of parental alleles in transgenic mice, *Nature* **328**:248–251.

Roberts, D. F., and Callow, M. H., 1980, Origin of the additional chromosome in Down's syndrome, *J. Med. Genet.* **39**:68–78.

Rothman, K. J., 1983, Spermicide use and Down's syndrome, *Am. J. Public Health* **72**:399–401.

Rowe, R. D., and Uchida, I. A., 1961, Cardiac malformations in mongolism: A prospective study of 184 mongoloid children, *Am. J. Med.* **31**:726.

Sacchi, N., Gusella, J. F., Perroni, L., Dagna Bricarelli, F., and Papas, T. S., 1988, Lack of evidence for association of meiotic nondisjunction with particular DNA haplotypes on chromosome 21, *Proc. Natl. Acad. Sci. USA* (in press).

Sandler, L., 1981, The meiotic nondisjunction of homologous chromosomes in *Drosophila* females, in: *Trisomy 21 (Down Syndrome): Research Perspectives* (F. de la Cruz and P. Gerald, eds.), pp. 181–197, University Park Press, Baltimore.

Sapienza, C., Peterson, A. C., Rossant, J., and Balling, R., 1987, Degree of methylation of transgenes is dependent on gamete of origin, *Nature* **328**:251–254.

Schweizer, D., Ambros, P., and Andrle, M., 1978, Modification of DAPI banding on human chromosomes by prestaining with a DNA-binding oligopeptide antibiotic, distamycin A, *Exp. Cell Res.* 111:327–332.

Searle, A. G., and Beechey, C., 1985, Noncomplementation phenomena and their bearing on nondisjunctional effects, in: *Aneuploidy, Etiology and Mechanisms* (V. L. Dellarco, P. E. Voytek, and A. Hollaender, eds.), pp. 363–276, Plenum Press, New York.

Shahar, S., and Morton, N. E., 1986, Origin of teratomas and twins, *Hum. Genet.* 74:215–218.

Shen, P., and Huang, H. V., 1986, Homologous recombination in *Escherichia coli:* Dependence on substrate length and homology, *Genetics* 11:441–457.

Slaugenhaupt, S. A., and Chakravarti, A., 1986, Methods for studying recombination on chromosomes that have undergone nondisjunction, *Am. J. Hum. Genet.* 39:168A.

Smith, G. E., and Berg, J. M., 1976, *Down's Anomaly,* Churchill Livingstone, Edinburgh.

Speed, R. M., 1977, The effects of aging on the meitoic chromosomes of male and female mice, *Chromosoma* 64:241–254.

Speed, R. M., and Chandley, A. C., 1983, Meiosis in the foetal mouse ovary. II. Oocyte development and age-related aneuploidy. Does a production line exist? *Chromosoma* 88:184–189.

Spinner, N. B., Eunpu, D. L., Schmickel, R. D., Zackai, E., Bunin, G., and Emanuel, B. S., 1986, The role of cytologic and molecular nor variants in trisomy 21, *Am. J. Hum. Genet.* 39(Suppl.):A133,392.

Stein, Z., Stein, W., and Susser, M., 1986, Attrition of trisomies as a maternal screening device, *Lancet* i:944–946.

Stewart, G. D., 1984, The isolation and characterisation of cloned DNA from a chromosome 21 enriched DNA library, Thesis, University of Glasgow, Scotland.

Stewart, G. D., Harris, P., Galt, J., and Ferguson-Smith, M. A., 1985, Cloned DNA probes regionally mapped to human chromosome 21 and their use in determining the origin of nondisjunction, *Nucleic Acids Res.* 13:4125–4132.

Stewart, G. D., Hassold, T. J., Berg, A., Watkins, P., Tanzi, R., and Kurnit, D. M., 1988, Down syndrome: Studying nondisjunction and meiotic recombination using cytogenetic and molecular polymorphisms that span chromosome 21, *Am. J. Hum. Genet.* 42:227–236.

Strobino, B., Kline, J., Lai, A., Stein, Z., Susser, M., and Warburton, D., 1986, Vaginal spermicides and spontaneous abortion of known karyotype, *Am. J. Epidemiol.* 123:431–443.

Sugawara, S., and Mikamo, K., 1983, Absence of correlation between univalent formation and meiotic nondisjunction in the aged female Chinese hamster, *Cytogenet. Cell Genet.* 35:34–40.

Tandon, R., and Edwards, J. E., 1973, Cardiac malformations associated with Down syndrome, *Circulation* 47:1349.

Tantravahi, U., Stewart, G. D., Roy, S., McNeil, G., Patterson, D., Van Keuren, M., Lalande, M., Kurnit, D. M., and Latt, S. A., 1988, Isolation of DNA sequences on chromosome 21 by application of a recombination-based assay to DNA from flow sorted chromosomes, *Hum. Genet.* (in press).

Tanzi, R. E., Haines, J. L., Stewart, G. D., Watkins, P. C., Gibbons, K. T., Faryniarz, A. G., Wallace, M. R., Hallewell, R., Yount, E., Wexler, N. S., Conneally, P. M., and Gusella, J. F., 1988, Genetic linkage map of chromosome 21, manuscript submitted to *Genomics*.

Therman, E., Otto, P. G., and Shahidi, N. T., 1981, Mitotic recombination and segregation of satellites in Bloom's syndrome, *Chromosoma* **82**:627–636.

Uchida, I., 1979, Radiation-induced nondisjunction, *Environ. Health Perspect.* **31**:13–18.

Van Keuren, M. L., Watkins, P. C., Drabkin, H. A., Jabs, E. W., Gusella, J. F., and Patterson, D., 1986, Regional localization of DNA sequences on chromosome 21 using somatic cell hybrids, *Am. J. Hum. Genet.* **38**:793–804.

Vekemans, M. J., and Trasler, D., 1985, Maternal genes control the extent of *in utero* selection against trisomic embryos in the mouse, *Am. J. Hum. Genet.* **37**(Suppl.):A128,377.

Waalwijk, C., and Flavell, R. A., 1978, DNA methylation at a CCGG sequence in the large intron of the rabbit beta-globin gene: Tissue specific variations, *Nucleic Acids Res.* **5**:4631–4641.

Wagenbicher, P., Killan, W., Aett, A., and Schnedl, W., 1976, Origin of the extra chromosome no. 21 in Down's syndrome, *Hum. Genet.* **32**:13–16.

Warren, A. C., Chakravarti, AA, Wong, C., Slaugenhaupt, S. A., Halloran, S. L., Watkins, P. C., Metaxotou, C., and Antonarakis, S. E., 1987, Evidence for reduced recombination on the nondisjoined chromosomes 21 in Down syndrome, *Science* **237**:652–654.

Watkins, P. C., Tanzi, R. E., Gibbons, K. T., Tricoli, J. V., Landes, G., Eddy, R., Shows, T. B., and Gusella, J. F., 1985, Isolation of polymorphic DNA segments from chromosome 21, *Nucleic Acids Res.* **13**:6075–6088.

Watt, V. M., Ingles, C. J., Urdea, M. S., and Rutter, W. J., 1985, Homology requirements for recombination in *Escherichia coli*, *Proc. Natl. Acad. Sci. USA* **82**:4768–4772.

Willard, H. F., and Waye, J. S., 1987, Hierarchical order in chromosome-specific human alpha satellite DNA, *Trends Genet.* **3**:192–198.

Chapter 5

Molecular Genetics of Human Salivary Proteins and Their Polymorphisms

Edwin A. Azen
Laboratory of Genetics and Department of Medicine
University of Wisconsin
Madison, Wisconsin 53706

Nobuyo Maeda
Laboratory of Genetics
University of Wisconsin
Madison, Wisconsin 53706

INTRODUCTION

The whole human saliva is a complex fluid that is produced by specialized salivary glands. The three major salivary glands (submandibular, parotid, and sublingual) produce most of the saliva, but the small buccal glands also contribute a minor amount. The human saliva is an easily obtained source of many proteins that are useful for genetic analysis (Boackle and Suddick, 1980; Mason and Chisholm, 1975; Vining and McGinley, 1986). In particular, the parotid saliva component (collected with the Curby cup) has advantages over whole saliva, including more uniform composition, less enzymatic degradation of proteins, and absence of contamination with bacteria or food. Stimulated parotid saliva [150–264 mg/100 ml total protein (Daniels and Newbrun, 1966)] contains 25–35 proteins, which can be stained in acid polyacrylamide or SDS gels with Coomassie brilliant blue R-250. Amylase and proline-rich proteins (PRPs)

141

constitute most of the proteins. In particular, the PRPs represent about two-thirds of the parotid salivary proteins and show numerous polymorphisms (Bennick, 1982, 1987; Azen, 1988). Many enzymes, hormones, growth factors, immunoglobulins, serum components, and other proteins (as the B_{12}-binding R proteins) can also be detected in saliva.

The subject of salivary protein polymorphisms was extensively reviewed in the late 1970s (Azen, 1978a; Tan and Teng, 1979; Teng and Tan, 1979) and also recently (Azen, 1988; Bennick, 1987). Thus, in this review we will focus to a greater degree on the recent molecular genetic studies of salivary protein gene systems. However, we will also discuss each of the known salivary protein polymorphisms in a concise fashion.

In the first section we describe inherited variations of a variety of salivary proteins with special reference to population studies in different ethnic groups; these population studies are summarized in Table I. We then describe recent molecular genetic studies for several salivary protein gene systems. Extensive molecular genetic data are available for the PRP gene family (which codes for most of the parotid salivary proteins). These studies on PRPs include gene organization and localization, mRNA processing, posttranslation modifications, and molecular and linkage analyses of insertion/deletion-type polymorphisms. We then discuss the more limited molecular genetic data for other salivary proteins, such as the cystatin protein gene family, coding for cysteine protease inhibitors, the amylase gene family, coding for pancreatic and salivary amylases, and the statherin gene, coding for a protein important in modulating calcium homeostasis in the saliva. In this review we emphasize the usefulness and potential of salivary proteins and their genes for many types of genetic research.

SALIVARY PROTEIN POLYMORPHISMS

Many of these polymorphisms are useful for population studies because the polymorphic variants show striking racial differences

TABLE I. Gene Frequencies of Salivary Protein Polymorphisms in Different Populations

System	Reference	S^a	n	Amy_1^A	Others
(Amy_1) Amylase[b] [in alkaline PAGE]	Merritt and Karn (1977)	WS			
	Whites (America)		961	0.995	0.005
	Blacks (America)		208	0.961	0.039
	Ikemoto et al. (1987)	WS			
	Japanese (Japan)		529	0.988	0.013
	Minaguchi and Suzuki (1981)	PS			
	Whites (Japan)		96	1.000	—

System	Reference	S	n	Amy_1	Amy_2^2	Amy_3^3	Others
(Amy_1) [in isoelectric focusing gels][c]	De Soyza (1978)	WS					
	Whites (England)		160	0.891	0.069	0.038	0.00
	Pronk et al. (1984)	PS					
	Whites (Netherlands)		330	0.907	0.067	0.027	—
	Blacks (West Africa, Bozo)		71	0.875	0.015	—	0.101
	Blacks (Kenya)	WS	200	0.959	0.008	—	0.051
	Kühnl and Tischberger (1980)						
	Whites (Germany)		170	0.909	0.070	0.021	—
	Eckersall and Beeley (1981)	WS					
	Whites (Scotland)		368	0.933	0.044	—	0.067

(continued)

TABLE I. (Continued)

System	Reference	S	n	Con 1+	Con 1-
(Con 1)					
Concanavalin A	Azen and Yu (1984a)	PS			
	Whites (America)		134	0.396	0.604
	Chinese (America)		79	0.580	0.420
	Blacks (America)		74	0.581	0.419

System	Reference	S	n	Con 2+	Con 2-
(Con 2)					
Concanavalin A	Azen and Yu (1984a)	PS			
	Whites (America)		134	0.034	0.966
	Chinese (America)		79	0	1.000
	Blacks (America)		74	0.007	0.993

System	Reference	S	n	Db+
(Db)				
Double band[a]	Azen and Denniston (1974)	PS		
	Whites (America)		100	0.12
	Blacks (America)		100	0.56
	Chinese (America)		54	0.07
	Ikemoto et al. (1987)	PS		
	Japanese (Japan)		350	0.033
	Minaguchi and Suzuki (1981)	PS		
	Whites (Japan)		94	0.143

	S	n	Gl¹	Gl²	Gl³	Gl⁴	Gl⁰	Others
Pronk et al. (1984)								
Whites (Netherlands)	PS	100	0.19					
Blacks (Kenya)		200	0.55					
Yu et al. (1980)	PS							
Whites (America)		685	0.179					
(G1)	**S**	**n**	**Gl¹**	**Gl²**	**Gl³**	**Gl⁴**	**Gl⁰**	**Others**
Major salivary glycoprotein								
Azen et al. (1979)	S							
Whites (America)		143	0.742	0.040	0.155	0.017	0.046	—
Blacks (America)		82	0.459	0.050	0.337	0.044	0.110	—
Minaguchi et al. (1981b)	PS							
Japanese (Japan)		104	0.555	0.033	0.245	0.033	0.105	0.029
(Pa)	**S**	**n**	$Pa^{1(+)}$	$Pa^{2(+)}$				
Acidic protein[d]								
Friedman et al. (1975)	PS							
Whites (America)		330	0.21	—				
Blacks (America)		122	0.14	—				
Chinese (America)		6	0.42	—				
Azen (1977)	PS							
Whites (America)		101	0.208	0.005				

(continued)

TABLE I. (*Continued*)

System	Reference	S	n	$Pa^{1(+)}$	$Pa^{2(+)}$
	Yu et al. (1980)				
	Whites (America)	PS	685	0.211	—
	Ikemoto et al. (1987)				
	Japanese (Japan)	PS	554	0.221	
	Minaguchi and Suzuki (1981)	PS			
	Whites (Japan)		96	0.158	—
	Pronk et al. (1984)	PS			
	Whites (Netherlands)		100	0.12	—
	Blacks (Kenya)		200	0.18	—

System	Reference	S	n	Pb^1	Pb^2
(*Pb*)					
Parotid basic protein	Azen (1972)	PS			
	Whites (America)		101	0.995	0.005
	Blacks (America)		90	0.840	0.160
	Ikemoto et al. (1987)	PS			
	Japanese (Japan)		435	1.000	—
	Pronk et al. (1984)	PS			
	Whites (Netherlands)		110	1.000	—
	Blacks (West Africa, Bozo)		71	0.800	0.200
	Minaguchi and Suzuki (1981)	PS			
	Blacks (Kenya)		200	0.880	0.120
	Whites (Japan)		91	1.000	—

	S	n	Pc^1	Pc^2
(Pc)				
Protein				
Karn et al. (1985)	PS			
Whites (America)		178	0.461	0.539
Blacks (America)		47	0.670	0.330

	S	n	Pe^+	Pe^-
(Pe)				
Protein				
Azen and Yu (1984b)	PS			
Whites (America)		317	0.76	0.24
Blacks (America)		51	0.76	0.24

	S	n	Ph^+	Ph^-
(Ph)				
Parotid heavy				
Ikemoto et al. (1987)	PS			
Japanese (Japan)		440	0.029	0.971
Minaguchi and Suzuki (1981)	PS			
Whites (Japan)		96	0	1.000
Noraini et al. (1980)	WS			
Malays (Malaysia)		147	0.082	0.918
Chinese (Malaysia)		189	0.109	0.891
Indians (Malaysia)		175	0.062	0.938

(continued)

TABLE I. (*Continued*)

System	Reference	S	n	PIF^+
(*PIF*)				
Parotid isoelectric focusing variant[d]	Azen and Denniston (1981)	PS		
	Whites (America)		148	0.66
	Blacks (America)		90	0.35
	Chinese (America)		78	0.56
	Ikemoto et al. (1987)	PS		
	Japanese (Japan)		257	0.721

System	Reference	S	n	Pm^+	Pm^-
(*Pm*) or *PmF*					
Parotid middle band, fast	Ikemoto et al. (1987)	PS			
	Japanese (Japan)		426	0.399	0.601
	Azen and Denniston (1980)	PS			
	Whites (America)		140	0.15	0.85
	Noraini et al. (1980)	WS			
	Malays (Malaysia)		172	0.385	0.615
	Chinese (Malaysia)		186	0.282	0.718
	Indians (Malaysia)		180	0.289	0.711
	Minaguchi and Suzuki (1981)	PS			
	Whites (Japan)		96	0.14	0.86

(PmS)

		n	PmS^+	PmS^-
Parotid middle band, slow				
Azen and Denniston (1980)	PS			
Whites (America)		140	0.12	0.88
Blacks (America)		101	0.24	0.76
Minaguchi and Suzuki[e]	PS			
Japanese (Japan)		254	0.354	0.646

(Po)

		n	Po^+	Po^-
Protein				
Azen and Yu (1984b)	PS			
Whites (America)		408	0.75	0.25
Blacks (America)		59	0.77	0.23

(Pr)

		n	Pr^1	Pr^2	$Pr^{1'}$
Proline-rich proteins					
Azen and Denniston (1974)	PS				
Whites (America)[f]		100	0.640	0.355	0.005
Blacks (America)[f]		100	0.700	0.250	0.050
Chinese (America)[f]		54	0.770	0.230	—
Ikemoto et al. (1987)	PS				
Japanese (Japan)		453	0.741	0.259	—

(continued)

TABLE I. (*Continued*)

System	Reference	S	n	Pr^1	Pr^2	$Pr^{1'}$
	Pronk et al. (1984)	PS				
	Whites (Netherlands)		100	0.81	0.19	—
	Blacks (Kenya)		200	0.66	0.34	—
	Minaguchi and Suzuki (1981)	PS				
	Whites (Japan)		95	0.721	0.279	—
	Yu et al. (1980)	PS				
	Whites (America)		685	0.718	0.282	

System	Reference	S	n	Ps^1	Ps^2	Ps^0	Others
(Ps)							
Parotid size variant	Azen and Denniston (1980)	PS					
	Whites (America)		150	0.598	0.101	0.301	—
	Blacks (America)		101	0.185	0.126	0.689	—
	Minaguchi et al. (1988)	PS					
	Japanese (Japan)		317	0.298	—	0.652	0.047

System	Reference	S	n	Rs^1	Rs^2
(Rs)					
B_{12}-binding R-proteins	Azen and Denniston (1979)	PS			
	Whites (America)		143	0.88	0.12
	Blacks (America)		104	0.94	0.06
	Chinese (America)		75	1.00	—
	Yang et al. (1982)	WS			
	Whites (America)		452	0.88	0.12

		n	Sal_I^F	Sal_I^1
Blacks (America)	S	48	0.99	0.01
Chinese (America)		136	1.00	—

(Sal_I) Proteins[g]

		n	Sal_I^F	Sal_I^1
Balakrishnan and Ashton (1974)	WS			
Whites (Hawaii)		154	0.403	0.597
Japanese (Hawaii)		42	0.364	0.636

(Sal_II) Proteins[g]

		n	Sal_{II}^S	Sal_{II}^1
Balakrishnan and Ashton (1974)	WS			
Whites (Hawaii)		154	0.573	0.427
Japanese (Hawaii)		42	0.591	0.409

(Sap_A) Acid phosphatase

		n	Sap_A^A	$Sap_A^{A'}$	Sap_A^0
Tan and Ashton (1976b)	WS				
Whites (Hawaii)		213	0.698	0.009	0.293
Japanese (Hawaii)		72	0.731	0.014	0.255

(continued)

TABLE I. (Continued)

System	Reference	S	n	Sap_B^B	Sap_B^0
(Sap_B) Acid phosphatase	Tan and Ashton (1976b)	WS			
	Whites (Hawaii)		213	0.773	0.227
	Japanese (Hawaii)		72	0.882	0.118

		S	n	$s\text{-}AcP^A$	$s\text{-}AcP^a$
($s\text{-}AcP$) Acid phosphatase	Ikemoto et al. (1985)	PS			
	Japanese (Japan)		183	0.227	0.773

		S	n	$SAPX^1$	$SAPX^2$	$SAPX^3$
($SAPX$) Salivary peroxidase	Azen (1977)	PS				
	Whites (America)		101	0.787	0.208	0.005
	Noraini et al. (1980)	WS				
	Malays (Malaysia)		143	0.762	0.238	
	Chinese (Malaysia)		151	0.755	0.245	
	Indians (Malaysia)		180	0.723	0.277	

		S	n	Sgd^1	Sgd^2
(Sgd)					
Glucose-6-phosphate dehydrogenase	Tan and Ashton (1976a)				
	Whites (Hawaii)	WS	190	0.755	0.245
	Japanese (Hawaii)		104	0.659	0.341

		S	n	Set_1^F	Set_1^S
(Set$_1$)					
Carboxylesterase	Tan (1976)				
	Whites (Hawaii)	WS	96	0.609	0.391
	Japanese (Hawaii)		53	0.500	0.500

[a] S, saliva source: WS is whole saliva; PS is parotid saliva.

[b] An extensive compilation of allelic frequencies of Amy tested by alkaline PAGE is presented by Merritt and Karn (1977).

[c] The nomenclature of Kühnl and Tischberger (1980) is used.

[d] Db, Pa, and PIF genetic determinants are expressed alleles without "nulls" at the PRH1 locus (Maeda, 1985; Azen et al., 1987).

[e] Personal communication.

[f] These data were recalculated by assuming that the phenotypes of all Pr 2' individuals are both Pr 2 and Pa$^+$.

[g] These polymorphisms studied in whole saliva are probably among acidic Pr proteins (Azen, 1978a).

in gene frequencies. The gene frequencies are given in Table I. Some of the more striking differences include: PIF^+ and Db^+ appear in much higher frequency in blacks compared to whites; Pb^2, $Pr^{1'}$, and some Amy variants are virtually confined to blacks; Pm^+ is more frequent in orientals than in whites; Gl^5 and Gl^6 occur in low frequencies in Japanese, but not in whites; the Rs^2 variant is commonly seen in whites, but not in Chinese.

Salivary Amylase (Amy)

Genetic variants detected by alkaline polyacrylamide slab gel electrophoresis were summarized by Merritt and Karn (1977). In whites, the combined frequency of these autosomal variants is low (less than 1%) and only reaches polymorphic proportions (7%) in blacks. However, Pronk (1977) and Pronk and Frants (1979) found, by isoelectric focusing in slab gels, two new alleles (Amy_1R^1 and Amy_1R^2) in the Dutch population, with frequencies of 0.06 and 0.03, respectively. These Amy variants are probably of the fast electrophoretic type, Amy_1R^1, as described by Merritt and Karn (1977), who recognized rare Amy_1R^1 homozygotes but could not resolve the more common heterozygote phenotypes. According to J. C. Pronk (personal communication), previously described amylase variants (Kamarýt and Laxová, 1966; Boettcher and de la Lande, 1969) are probably of the same general type as those described more recently by Pronk (1977). Similar observations were made by de Soyza (1978) in a white population by isoelectric focusing in slab gels, and six Amy phenotypes representing four alleles were described. Kühnl and Tischberger (1980) studied salivary amylase in a white population by isoelectric focusing in slab gels and found that the gene frequencies of the three common alleles were very similar to those recorded by Pronk and Frants (1979). Eckersall and Beeley (1981) described in a white population several amylase variants with combined frequency of 11.7%. They stained the isoelectric focusing gels with starch-iodine, which is more sensitive than protein staining for detecting amylase variants. Evidence for duplication of the human salivary amylase gene was provided by Pronk et al. (1982), based on analysis of a puzzling electrophoretic pattern interpreted to represent three different amylase gene products in each of four individuals. The biochemical basis of the variant phenotypes has not been determined, but their polymorphic frequencies extend the usefulness of salivary amylase for further genetic studies.

B_{12}-Binding Protein (Rs)

There are three classes of human B_{12}-binding proteins: gastric intrinsic factor, which facilitates B_{12} absorption from the small intestine; plasma transcobalamin II (TC II), which facilitates cellular uptake of B_{12} by tissues; and R-proteins, which are found in several body fluids and tissues. The R-proteins may subserve antibacterial, transport, or protective binding functions. As summarized by Allen (1975), all R-proteins share a common protein backbone and differ among each other only in the amount and proportion of attached carbohydrates. Also, these three classes of B_{12} binding proteins are probably products of three genes.

Azen and Denniston (1979) found in parotid saliva a polymorphism of B_{12}-binding R-proteins, and the polymorphism (termed Rs) is determined by autosomal inheritance of two codominant alleles. The polymorphism was revealed by neuraminidase treatment and radiolabeling ($^{57}CoB_{12}$) of the R-proteins in parotid saliva followed by isoelectric focusing of the proteins in slab gels (pH 4–6.5). The Rs polymorphism is shared by B_{12}-binding R-proteins of milk, tears, and leukocytes. Daiger et al. (1978) and Fráter-Schröeder et al. (1979) found genetic polymorphism of the plasma B_{12}-binder TC II. However, there is no evidence for close linkage between Rs and TC II or between Rs and several PRP genetic determinants (Azen and Denniston, 1979). Yang et al. (1982) used similar methods in a later study and found the same polymorphism as Rs in whole saliva and granulocytes. Carmel and Herbert (1969) described a family in which two brothers had congenital absence of R-type binders of vitamin B_{12} in serum, saliva, cerebrospinal fluid, gastric juice, and granulocytes. The saliva contained no immunological R-binder, but cross-reacting material was found in serum. There was no clinical abnormality due to the defect.

Salivary Acid Phosphatase (s-AcP)

Genetic polymorphism of human parotid salivary acid phosphate (s-AcP) was described in a Japanese population by Ikemoto *et al.* (1985), who separated the proteins in pH 4.0–6.5 isoelectric focusing slab gels. Two codominant alleles at an autosomal locus determined three variant protein patterns. The relationship of this polymorphism to that described in whole saliva by Tan and Ashton (1976*b*) is unclear.

Genetic Polymorphisms of Proline-Rich Proteins (PRPs)

General Features of PRPs

We will first discuss the general features of the PRPs and their polymorphisms and then give a brief description of each of the polymorphisms. About 70% of the proteins of human saliva are PRPs, and proline alone accounts for 25–40% of the amino acids (Bennick, 1982). Proline, glycine, and glutamine (glutamic acid) together constitute 70–80% of amino acids of PRPs. The PRPs can be subdivided into three groups: glycosylated, basic, and acidic, accounting for approximately 17, 23, and 30%, respectively, of the total protein in parotid saliva, although there is some overlap between glycosylated and basic PRPs. The PRPs have also been found in acinic cell carcinomas of the parotid salivary glands (Warner *et al.*, 1985) and in serous cells of the submucosal glands of the respiratory tract (Warner and Azen, 1984; Ito *et al.*, 1985). Tooth-related functions [reviewed by Bennick (1982)] have been assigned to acidic PRPs: they bind to calcium and maintain it in the supersaturated state (thus avoiding calcium precipitation in salivary ducts or in the oral cavity); they form a part of the dental pellicle; and they bind to hydroxyapatite. Since PRPs are found in serous cells of the submucosal glands of the respiratory tract, they may subserve other functions, such as effects on viscosity. The production of PRPs is stimulated in the rat and mouse by feeding sorghums containing high levels of tannins (Mehansho *et al.*, 1983, 1985). Tannins are known to be toxic and carcinogenic, and bind strongly to salivary PRPs. Therefore, it was proposed that salivary PRPs may tightly bind tannins and thus protect dietary proteins, digestive enzymes, and the gastrointestinal tract from these detrimental effects (Mehansho et al., 1987). Salivary PRPs might also protect the esophagus from the carcinogenic influence of tannins (Warner and Azen, 1988). Genes for PRPs and bitter taste are closely linked in the mouse (Azen et al., 1986); however, there is no direct evidence that PRPs subserve specific taste functions.

The many PRPs show complex electrophoretic patterns and marked variations in different individuals. These variations are due to numerous genetic polymorphisms and associated posttranslational processes, such as proteolysis. Four polymorphisms for acidic PRPs include Pr [proline-rich (Azen and Oppenheim, 1973; Azen and Denniston, 1974)], Pa [acidic protein (Friedman et al., 1975; Azen, 1977, 1978a)], Db [double band (Azen and Denniston, 1974)], and PIF [parotid isoelectric-focusing variant (Azen and Denniston, 1981)]. Eight polymorphisms for basic and glycosylated PRPs are Pm [parotid middle band (Ikemoto et al., 1977)], PmS [parotid middle slow band (Azen and Denniston, 1980)], Ps [parotid size variant (Azen and Denniston, 1980)], G1 [major glycoprotein (Azen et al., 1979)], Con 1 and Con 2 [concanavalin A binding (Azen and Yu, 1984a)], Po (Azen and Yu, 1984b), and Pc (Karn et al., 1985). Polymorphism for the almost neutral Pe protein has also been described (Azen and Yu, 1984b).

Several different terminologies were applied to the PRPs by different workers, who were interested primarily in genetic or biochemical characterizations. Thus, Anderson et al. (1982a) found that the PmS polymorphic protein is the same as the basic PRP IB-6 [P-I of Saitoh et al. (1983b)] and the PmF polymorphic protein is the same as the basic PRP IB-9 [P-E of Isemura et al. (1982)]. Also, Azen and Oppenheim (1973) established the identity of the polymorphic acidic Pr proteins 1–4 with purified PRPs I–IV (Oppenheim et al., 1971). Among other acidic PRPs, the PIF polymorphic proteins were probably inadvertently copurified with acidic PRPs C and A (Azen and Denniston, 1981; E. A. Azen and A. Bennick, unpublished; Maeda et al., 1985), and Db and Pa polymorphic proteins may be among other acidic PRPs described by Hay and Oppenheim (1974). To further match polymorphic PRPs with other biochemically purified PRPs, a number of purified PRPs, provided by E. Saitoh, D. Kauffman, and P. Keller, were electrophoretically compared in more than one gel system with polymorphic PRPs in parotid saliva (Azen, 1988). These electrophoretic identities will be noted as each polymorphism is discussed. Among the PRP polymorphisms, only Ps, Con 1, and Con 2 proteins could not be electrophoretically identified with the available purified PRPs.

The PRP polymorphisms show several unusual phenotypes, which include double-banded patterns among the acidic PRPs, molecular size variants, and frequent null (unexpressed) forms. The electrophoretic methods and characteristic polymorphic phenotypes of PRPs in several gel systems were recently summarized (Azen, 1988). We now discuss these unusual phenotypic features. The first PRP polymorphism described was that termed Pr (Azen and Oppenheim, 1973; Azen and Denniston, 1974); each Pr allele determines a double-banded phenotype. The three alleles (*Pr* 1, *Pr* 1', and *Pr* 2) at an autosomal locus account for the variant double-banded phenotypes (Azen and Denniston, 1974). The allele termed *Pr* 2' (Azen and Denniston, 1974) was later found to be the *Pr* 2 allele associated with the *Pa*$^+$ allele (Azen, 1977). Therefore, the designation *Pr* 2' is no longer appropriate. The double-banded pattern of the Pr proteins is due to partial proteolytic cleavage. Thus, Karn *et al.* (1979) found that the smaller Pr 3 and Pr 4 proteins are derived from the larger Pr 1 and Pr 2 proteins, respectively, by posttranslational cleavages by a salivary protease. The amino acid sequences of protein A (Pr 3) and protein C (Pr 1) were determined by Wong *et al.* (1979) and Wong and Bennick (1980), who found the sequence of protein A to be identical to the N-terminal 106 residues of protein C, which is 150 residues in length. Wong *et al.* (1983) subsequently found that the protease kallikrein, derived from saliva, could cleave protein C (Pr 1) on the carboxyl side of Arg-106 *in vitro*. The salivary peptide P-C (Isemura *et al.,* 1980) is identical to the C-terminal 44 residues of protein C (Pr 1) and represents the smaller of the two cleavage products. However, Wong *et al.* (1983) found no evidence that the proteolytic cleavage by kallikrein occurs primarily in the saliva or salivary ducts, implying that this process occurs mainly in the acinar cells of the gland.

The acidic PRPs, PIF (Azen and Denniston, 1981) and Db (Azen and Denniston, 1974), also show double-banded patterns, and the smaller protein is probably generated from the larger one by proteolytic cleavage at Arg-106. There is strong evidence for this, since, from DNA analysis, both PIF and Db proteins possess the Arg-106 residue (Maeda *et al.*, 1985; Azen *et al.*, 1987).

The Pa protein is probably not cleaved by proteolysis, since the acidic Pa protein polymorphism (unlike the Pr, Db, and PIF polymorphisms) shows only a single-banded rather than a double-banded pattern. The Pa protein (unlike other PRPs) is probably a dimer and contains cysteine residues (Goodman *et al.*, 1985; Azen *et al.*, 1987) with a disulfide linkage between monomeric subunits (Azen, 1977, 1978*a*).

Allelic variants of two basic PRP polymorphisms (G1 and Ps) are unusual, since they are characterized by molecular size rather than the usual charge differences (Azen *et al.*, 1979; Azen and Denniston, 1980). The findings (to be discussed later) of tandem repeats in the PRPs suggest that unequal crossing over at the gene level might lead to deletions and duplications of DNA in coding regions, with consequent protein size differences.

All of the PRP polymorphisms, with the exception of Pr and Pc, show null phenotypes, i.e., apparent lack of protein expression in saliva. The molecular basis for the frequent null phenotypes among PRPs is now better understood and will be discussed later. To summarize, among basic PRPs, null phenotypes are due, in some cases (e.g., PmS and PmF), to genetic variations at proteolytic cut sites (Lyons *et al.*, 1988*b*). The acidic PRPs, Pa, Db, and PIF, are now known to be determined by alleles (without nulls) at a single locus (*PRH1*) rather than by three separate loci (Maeda, 1985; Azen *et al.*, 1987). Numerous family linkage studies based on the protein polymorphisms and summarized by Goodman *et al.* (1985) indicate that the PRPs are determined by a closely linked, multigene family (on a single autosome), which may span 15 map units. Additionally, many studies [summarized by Goodman *et al.* (1985)] show nonrandom associations between phenotypes of different protein polymorphisms. The exact nature of these associations is unknown, although in some cases linkage disequilibrium (related to closely linked genes) may be occurring. Also, as will be discussed later, PmF and PmS, which show strong associations, are both processed from the same gene transcript (Lyons *et al.*, 1988*b*). Some striking associations are shown in Table II between PmS and PmF; Con 2 and PmF; and Pa$^+$ and Pr 2.

Based on biochemical studies of PRPs, one can say that the PRP multigene family probably evolved by a process of gene duplication, since the various PRPs are closely related. Thus, from many studies, the various PRPs are strikingly similar in amino acid composition and amino acid sequence. Thus, with one exception, the first 54 residues in the amino acid sequences of IB-9 (PmF) and IB-6 (PmS) are identical (Kauffman *et al.*, 1982); also, IB-1 and IB-6 contain an identical sequence of 54 residues except for one residue (Kauffman *et al.*, 1986). There is also considerable homology between the amino acid sequences of IB-9 and IB-6 and the C-terminal portion of the acidic PRP protein C. Other interesting amino acid sequence homologies among acidic and basic PRPs are summarized by Bennick (1987). From amino acid sequence data (Wong and Bennick, 1980; Kauffman *et al.*, 1982; Saitoh *et al.*, 1983*a*; Kauffman *et al.*, 1986), there are frequent and similar tandem repeats in different PRPs. Also, Azen and Denniston (1980) showed extensive immunological cross-reactivity between many different PRPs. Therefore, the hypothesized process of gene duplication within the PRP gene family may have occurred in part through unequal crossing over, facilitated by the similar tandem repeats.

PRP Polymorphisms

Proline-Rich Acidic Proteins (Pr). This was the first of the PRP polymorphisms described in parotid saliva (Azen and Oppenheim, 1973). These early studies detailed the autosomal codominant inheritance of two proteins (Pr 1 and 3) determined by gene *Pr*^{1} and two other proteins (Pr 2 and 4) determined by the gene *Pr*^{2}. It is now known (as discussed before) that the smaller Pr 3 and Pr 4

TABLE II. Positive Associations (Observed/Expected) in Randomly Collected Parotid Saliva Samples from Whites[a]

	Pa+	Pa-	Total		Con 2+	Con 2-	Total		PmS+	PmS-	Total
Pr 2 types / PmF+	37 / 13.9	0 / 23.1	37		9 / 2.3	25 / 31.7	34		25 / 6.5	9 / 27.5	34
Other Pr types / PmF-	1 / 24.1	63 / 39.9	64		0 / 6.7	100 / 98.3	100		0 / 18.5	96 / 77.5	96
Total	38	63	101		9	125	134		25	105	130

$\chi^2 = 92.7, p < 0.0001$ $\chi^2 = 24.31, p < 0.0001$ $\chi^2 = 82.7, p < 0.0001$

[a] Association data are from the following sources: Pa/Pr (Azen, 1977); Con 2/PmF and PmS/PmF (Azen and Yu, 1984a).

proteins are derived from the larger Pr 1 and Pr 2 proteins by proteolysis. The Pr proteins 1–4 are easily separated in the alkaline polyacrylamide gel system and appear as double-banded patterns, but the single-banded Pa protein may overlap the uncommon Pr 1' protein characteristic of Pr 1' types seen mostly in blacks (Azen and Denniston, 1974; Azen, 1977, 1978a). However, the Pr 1' protein can be easily separated from the Pa protein in isoelectric focusing slab gels (Azen and Denniston, 1981). The polymorphic proteins Pr 1–4 are identical to the four classic Pr proteins (Pr I–IV) partially characterized by Oppenheim et al. (1971), and Pr 1 and Pr 3 are the same as protein C and protein A, respectively, as characterized by Bennick and colleagues (Bennick, 1982). The isoelectric points of the Pr proteins range from 4.09 to 4.71, and the molecular weights of proteins C and A are approximately 16,500 and 11,700, respectively. E. Azen and G. Larson (unpublished) gel-purified the Pr 1' protein and compared its size to that of the Pr 1 protein by SDS gel electrophoresis. The Pr 1' protein is the same size as the Pr 1 protein; therefore, the electrophoretic difference between Pr 1' and Pr 1 proteins in nondenaturing gel systems (Azen and Denniston, 1974, 1981; Azen, 1978a) is more likely to be due to a charge than to a size difference. The Pr 1' phenotype is double-banded, and the larger cleaved product shows the same mobility as Pr 3 in nondenaturing gels. Therefore, we suspect that the presumed charge difference between the Pr 1' and Pr 1 proteins resides in the smaller "P-C-like" cleavage product (not seen on the gel).

The acidic PRPs (Pr, Db, Pa, and PIF) show unusual staining properties. They stain intensely blue with "stains all" (Azen, 1978a) in alkaline gels and negatively against a dark background with 3-3' dimethoxybenzidine (Azen and Oppenheim, 1973; Azen and Denniston, 1974). They can be stained for phosphate after alkaline hydrolysis (Azen, 1978b) and show an unusual pink-violet color when stained with Coomassie brilliant blue R-250 in a solution of methanol–water–acetic acid (Henkin et al., 1978; Azen and Yu, 1984b). However, routinely most PRPs are readily identified by staining with Coomassie brilliant blue R-250 in the presence of trichloracetic acid. To summarize, there are three identified Pr alleles without nulls (Pr

1, *Pr* 2, and *Pr* 1') at a locus now termed *PRH*2 to be discussed later (Maeda, 1985; Azen *et al.*, 1987).

Acidic Protein (Pa). Friedman *et al.* (1975) described polymorphism of a parotid protein termed the "Pa 1 protein" (acidic protein), which was detected using starch gel electrophoresis and a stain for arginine-rich proteins (Sung and Smithies, 1969). The common Pa 1 protein is either present or absent from all saliva samples and shows autosomal inheritance. Subsequently Azen (1977) identified a rare variant termed Pa 2. The Pa genetic determinant was shown to be closely linked to the PRP multigene locus by family protein studies (Goodman *et al.*, 1985). Friedman *et al.* (1975) showed that the Pa 1 protein is similar in amino acid composition to the Pr (proline-rich) proteins characterized by Oppenheim *et al.* (1971) with an isoelectric point in the range of 3.9–4.5, but with a larger molecular weight than the Pr proteins. This molecular weight difference was confirmed by a study of Pr and Pa proteins in alkaline slab polyacrylamide gels (Azen, 1977). Although Friedman *et al.* (1975) reported no cysteine in the composition of the Pa 1 protein, Azen (1977, 1978*a*), employing disulfide-splitting agents and ^{14}C-labeled iodoacetamide to identify monomeric products, showed that the Pa 1 protein is a dilsulfide-bonded dimer. In a later study, amino acid analysis showed a single cysteine per monomer subunit in the Pa protein (Goodman *et al.*, 1985). The Pa 1 protein probably complexes with salivary lactoperoxidase through disulfide bond formation (Azen, 1977), and this will be discussed later.

Although the Pr, PIF, and Db acidic proteins show double-banded electrophoretic phenotypes, the Pa protein appears as a single band in several gel systems (summarized by Azen, 1988). As will be discussed later, the *Pa* genetic determinant is now known to be allelic to *Db* and *PIF* at a single locus termed *PRH*1 (Maeda, 1985; Azen *et al.*, 1987). The single-banded pattern is due to a cysteine substitution in the 150-amino acid subunit at Arg-103 near the Arg-106 proteolytic cut site, and this may present partial proteolysis that probably accounts for the double-banded patterns of Pr, Db, and PIF acidic proteins. Phenotypically, the Pa protein is strongly associated with Pr 2 proteins (Table II).

Double-Band Proteins (Db). This pair of acidic proteins, found in parotid saliva and termed Db, is identified in several gel systems (Azen and Denniston, 1974, 1981; Azen, 1978a), and is autosomally inherited. From early family protein studies of Azen and Denniston (1974), *Db* was shown to be closely linked to the *Pr* locus. The pair of Db proteins is either present or absent from all salivas (Azen and Denniston, 1974). As noted previously, the double-banded electrophoretic pattern can be explained by partial proteolysis of the 150-amino acid protein at the Arg-106 cut site. As will be discussed later, the *Db* genetic determinant is allelic to *Pa* and *PIF* at a locus termed *PRH1* (Maeda, 1985; Azen et al., 1987). Its primary structure is 21 amino acids longer than the equal-sized Pa monomer and PIF proteins (Azen et al., 1987).

Parotid Isoelectric Focusing Variant (PIF). Azen and Denniston (1981) found this genetic polymorphism among parotid salivary proteins. The polymorphism is detected after separation in pH 3.5–5.2 urea isoelectric focusing slab gels and staining with Coomassie brilliant blue R-250, or more conveniently by simply precipitating the proteins in the slab gel with trichloracetic acid. The autosomally inherited phenotypes show a pair of bands (PIF S and PIF F) that are either present or absent from all salivas. The genetic determinant for the PIF proteins is closely linked to that for *Gl*, which codes for the major glycoprotein, a known PRP (Azen and Denniston, 1981). As will be discussed later, the cDNA for the PIF protein has been isolated, and its structure is that of an acidic PRP determined by the *PRH1* locus (Maeda et al., 1985). Also, the PIF F (fast) protein is derived from the PIF S (slow) protein by post-translational proteolytic cleavege at the Arg-106 cut site, and *PIF* is allelic to *Db* and *Pa* at the *PRH1* locus (Maeda 1985; Azen et al., 1987). The PIF S and PIF F proteins have isoelectric points that are very close to those for the acidic PRPs, Pr 1 (protein C) and Pr 3 (protein A), respectively. Therefore, as noted by Azen and Denniston (1981), the PIF and Pr proteins (C and A) would have been difficult to separate during previous attempts at purification of Pr proteins (Bennick, 1977). Indeed, the PIF proteins were inadvertently copurified with acidic PRPs C and A (Maeda et al., 1985; Bennick, 1987; E. A. Azen and A. Bennick, unpublished results).

Fast Parotid Middle Band (PmF). Ikemoto et al. (1977) described the Pm basic protein polymorphism in parotid saliva. This polymorphism was detected after electrophoresis in starch gels that were stained for arginine-rich proteins (Sung and Smithies, 1969). The polymorphism is autosomally inherited as a protein that is either present or absent from all salivas. Minaguchi *et al.* (1981*a*) found the amino acid composition of the Pm protein to be typical for that of a PRP. The Pm(PmF) protein is electrophoretically the same (Azen, 1988) as PRP IB-9 of Kauffman and Keller (1979) and P-E of Isemura *et al.* (1982).

Slow Parotid Middle Band (PmS).   Azen and Denniston (1980) described genetic polymorphism of the PmS basic protein in acid polyacrylamide slab gels stained with Coomassie brilliant blue R-250. The polymorphism is autosomally inherited, and is either present or absent from all salivas. Phenotypically, it is closely associated with the smaller Pm(PmF) protein described by Ikemoto *et al.* (1977). Thus, the PmS + type is always associated with PmF + , and the PmS − type is almost always associated with PmF − , but sometimes is associated with PmF + (Table II). The PmF and PmS proteins are now known to be processed products of a single PRP gene termed *PRB1* (Lyons *et al.*, 1988*b*). The Pm genetic determinants are closely linked to those for other PRPs (Azen and Denniston, 1980; Goodman *et al.*, 1985), and the Pm proteins are immunologically related to other PRPs (Azen and Denniston, 1980). The PmS protein is electrophoretically the same (Azen, 1988) as the PRPs IB-6 of Kauffman and Keller (1979) and P-I of Saitoh *et al.* (1983*b*). However, biochemically there are unresolved amino acid differences between PRPs IB-6 and P-I (D. Kauffman and P. Keller, personal communication). The primary amino acid sequences of IB-6 and IB-9 were determined by Kauffman *et al.* (1982, 1986).

Major Parotid Salivary Glycoprotein (G1).   The major parotid salivary glycoprotein contains about 40% carbohydrate, is rich in proline, glycine, and glutamic acid, has an isoelectric point of greater than pH 8.2, and has a molecular weight of around 36,000. Levine *et al.* (1969) state that this glycoprotein accounts for 21–25% of stimulated parotid salivary proteins and 75% of the total carbohydrate. Azen *et al.* (1979) described genetic polymorphisms of G1 in parotid saliva after electrophoresis of the proteins in acid polyacylamide slab gels and staining with the periodic acid-Schiff reagent for glycoproteins. G1 is the same as the IA glycoprotein of Kauffman and Keller (1979). The CD-IIf peptide of Shimomura *et al.* (1983) is found within the G1 protein. The G1 polymorphism is determined by autosomal inheritance of at least four expressed alleles and one unexpressed allele in blacks and whites. Minaguchi *et al.* (1981*b*) studied a Japanese population for G1 variants and they found two new, very slow migrating variants in acid polyacrylamide slab gels. This will be discsussed later with relationship to the Ph protein polymorphism. From early family studies (Azen *et al.*, 1979), there is close linkage of *G1* to other PRP genetic determinants. This represented evidence that the closely linked, multigene PRP family includes genetic determinants for basic as well as acidic PRPs and strongly suggested that genes determining other salivary PRPs would also be linked to the same gene family. Amino acid compositions of G1 1 and G1 4 variant proteins strongly resemble the compositions of the major basic glycoprotein and acidic PRPs described by others (Azen *et al.*, 1979). The G1 protein polymorphism is determined by apparent differences in molecular weights of the variant proteins. This is an unusual finding, since most previously described protein polymorphisms are due to charge differences. The G1 proteins are now known to be products of the PRP gene termed *PRB3* (Lyons *et al.*, 1988*b*).

Salivary Parotid Heavy Protein (Ph). Genetic polymorphism of a large glycoprotein was described by Ikemoto *et al.* (1979) in a Japanese population, and the polymorphism was detected in SDS–urea gels stained with Coomassie brilliant blue. The polymorphism is autosomally inherited and the protein is either present or absent from all salivas. Since the Ph and G1 proteins are of similar molecular size in SDS gels and since both are well stained for carbohydrate with the periodic acid-Schiff reagent, it is likely that the Ph protein is an allelic form of the G1 protein. In support of this, Minaguchi *et al.* (1981*b*) found two very slowly migrating G1 variant proteins in the acid polyacrylamide gel system in Japanese, but not in whites. It is thus likely that one or both of the G1 variants might represent the Ph protein(s), since the Ph + variant (like the slow G1 variants) was also not seen in whites (Minaguchi and Suzuki, 1981).

Parotid Size Variant (Ps).   Azen and Denniston (1980) described genetic polymorphisms of the basic Ps proteins in acid polyacrylamide slab gels stained with Coomassie brilliant blue R-250. As with G1, this polymorphism is characterized by apparent differences in molecular weights in acid polyacrylamide and SDS gels. Goodman and Karn (1983) confirmed these molecular weight differences by subjecting purified Ps proteins to limited proteolysis with several enzymes. Digestion patterns indicate considerable homology between Ps isoproteins.

The Ps polymorphism is autosomally inherited as expressed and unexpressed alleles. In the initial report, only two expressed alleles were found, but Minaguchi *et al.* (1988) later found, in a Japanese population, evidence for other Ps variants. There is close linkage between *Ps* and other genetic determinants for PRPs (Azen and Denniston, 1980; Goodman *et al.*, 1985). From amino acid analysis, the Ps proteins have the typical amino acid composition of the PRP family (Goodman *et al.*, 1985). Also, Ps proteins cross-react immunologically with other PRPs when tested with antisera to several specific PRPs (Azen and Denniston, 1980). The Ps proteins are probably products of the PRP gene termed *PRB2* (Lyons *et al.*, 1988*b*).

Concanavalin A-Binding Proteins (Con 1 and Con 2).   Azen and Yu (1984*a*) found in parotid saliva two basic protein polymorphisms (Con 1 and Con 2), each of which is autosomally determined and is either present or absent from all salivas. The Con proteins are typed after transfers to nitrocellulose from SDS gels and identification with peroxidase-labeled concanavalin A. The genetic determinants for these proteins are tightly linked to those for other PRPs, and the Con proteins cross-react immunologically with other PRPs when tested with antisera to several specific PRPs (Azen and Yu, 1984*a*). Phenotypically, the Con 2 protein is strongly associated with the Pm(PmF) protein (Table II). The Con 1 and Con 2 proteins are probably products of the PRP gene, termed *PRB4*, and the glycopeptide, CD-IIg of Shimomura *et al.* (1983), is also coded by *PRB4* (Lyons *et al.*, 1988*b*).

Pe Protein.   This polymorphism, found in parotid saliva by Azen and Yu (1984*b*), is autosomally determined and is either present or absent from all salivas. The Pe protein polymorphism is typed in alkaline polyacrylamide slab gels stained with Coomassie brilliant blue R-250. The genetic determinant for Pe is probably closely linked to those of other PRPs, and the Pe protein cross-reacts immunologically with other PRPs (Azen and Yu, 1984*b*). The Pe protein is electrophoretically the same (Azen, 1988) as the DEAEII-2 PRP of Kauffman and Keller (1979) and it has an isoelectric point of approximately pH 6.1–6.3 (Azen and Yu, 1984*b*). This isoelectric point is unusual for a PRP, which is usually much more basic or acidic. The Pe protein is a product of the PRP gene termed *PRB1* (Lyons *et al.*, 1988*b*).

Po Protein.   This basic protein polymorphism (Azen and Yu, 1984*b*), found in parotid saliva, is autosomally determined and is either present or absent from all salivas. The polymorphism is typed by immunological reactivity to anti-PRP serum or by protein staining after transfers to nitrocellulose from SDS gels. The genetic determinant for Po is closely linked to those of other PRPs. The Po protein is electrophoretically the same (Azen, 1988) as the PRPs IB-5 (Kauffman and Keller, 1979) and P-D (Saitoh *et al.*, 1983*c*). However, biochemically there are unresolved amino acid differences between PRPs IB-5 and P-D (D. L. Kauffman and P. J. Keller, personal communication). The Po protein is a product of the PRP gene termed *PRB4* (Lyons *et al.*, 1988*b*).

Pc Protein.   Karn *et al.* (1985) described this polymorphism in parotid saliva, and it is autosomally determined by two expressed alleles. The polymorphism is typed after electrophoresis and protein staining in acid polyacrylamide slab gels, and the proteins immunologically cross-react with the Pr 1 and Ps 1 proteins by Ouchterlony analysis when tested against an antiserum to whole parotid salivary proteins. The amino acid compositions of the Pc proteins are very similar to those of other basic PRPs (Karn *et al.*, 1985), and by electrophoretic analysis (Azen, 1988), the Pc protein is the same as the IB-8a PRP of Kauffman and Keller (1979). There is suggestive but not conclusive evidence of linkage of the Pc genetic determinant to those of other PRPs (Karn *et al.*, 1985). The Pc protein has not yet been assigned to a specific PRP gene.

Salivary Peroxidase (SAPX)

Azen (1977) found in parotid saliva genetic variants of SAPX with different electrophoretic mobilities in acid polyacrylamide slab gels stained with p-phenylenediamine and hydrogen peroxide. The two most common genetic types are SAPX-1 and SAPX-2; an uncommon type (SAPX 3) was also found. There is strong (although not conclusive) evidence that the electrophoretically larger forms of SAPX (SAPX 2 and SAPX 3) represent modified forms of the smaller SAPX 1. First, family data indicate completely codominant expression of SAPX 2 and SAPX 3 types, whereas the SAPX 1 type shows recessive inheritance. Second, the presumed modified forms of SAPX (SAPX 2 and SAPX 3) show larger molecular weights then the presumed unmodified form (SAPX 1). Third, the larger molecular weight forms (SAPX 2 and SAPX 3) can be converted to the smaller form (SAPX 1) by splitting disulfide bonds, perhaps dissociating a disulfide-bonded complex between SAPX 1 and another molecule.

Surprisingly, when saliva samples were typed for both Pa and SAPX protein polymorphisms, there was a perfect correspondence between Pa and SAPX types. Thus, the presence of the Pa protein in either its common form (Pa 1) or much less common form (Pa 2) correlates perfectly with "modified" SAPX types (SAPX 2 and SAPX 3). Alternatively, the absence of Pa proteins correlates perfectly with the presence of the "unmodified" SAPX 1 type.

As noted in the discussion previously, the Pa protein is a disulfide-bonded dimer with one cysteine per subunit. Thus, it is postulated that SAPX 2 and SAPX 3 types are probably complexes of SAPX 1 with Pa 1 and Pa 2 thiol monomers, respectively, through disulfide bond formation. However, it will be necessary to characterize the SAPX types biochemically in order to prove or disprove this modification hypothesis.

Many studies note the occurrence and significance in saliva of an antibacterial system consisting of peroxidase, thiocyanate (SCN^-), and hydrogen peroxide (Tenovuo and Pruitt, 1984). Therefore, does the occurrence of genetic variants of SAPX proteins in saliva have any biological or clinical significance as considered by

Azen (1985)? As a first step in answering this question, SAPX enzyme activities were assessed in salivas of SAPX 1 and SAPX 2 types using a *p*-phenylenediamine substrate (Azen, 1978*c*). There were no significant differences in SAPX enzyme activities in the two groups. In clinical studies of children, Yu *et al.* (1986) have shown that the Pa + phenotype (always associated with the complexed form of SAPX) is correlated with an increase in DMFS (decayed–missing–filled tooth surface) score as compared to the Pa – phenotype (always associated with the unmodified SAPX). Other studies, however, show no correlation of PRP phenotypes or levels of acidic PRPs to dental disease (Anderson *et al.*, 1982*b*; Anderson and Mandel, 1982; Mandel and Bennick, 1983).

Parotid Basic Proteins (Pb)

Azen (1972) described polymorphism of these basic small-molecular weight proteins among blacks. The proteins represent the most rapidly migrating components in acid urea starch gels stained for arginine-rich proteins (Sung and Smithies, 1969). The unusual phenotypes show a peculiar asymmetry of alternative homozygous types and are the expression of two alleles, Pb^1 and Pb^2. The Pb 1 homozygote shows four electrophoretic bands (a, b, d, and e), whereas the less common Pb 2 homozygote shows only one band (c), which differs in mobility from the other bands. Also, there are slight variations in mobility and intensity of Pb bands in samples of the same phenotype. Proteolytic degradation of Pb proteins occurring in the parotid gland probably causes these variations within phenotypes (Azen, 1972, 1973).

The Pb proteins are among the "histidine-rich" proteins that have been isolated from saliva by several groups of workers (Balekjian and Longton, 1973; Hay, 1975; Baum *et al.*, 1976; Holbrook and Molan, 1975; MacKay *et al.*, 1984*a*). Oppenheim *et al.* (1986) isolated the neutral, histidine-rich polypeptide from parotid saliva and determined its primary structure. The amino acid sequence, although related, is significantly different from that of other histidine-rich peptides such as Pb and PPb (to be discussed later).

Hay (1975) found a salivary histidine-rich peptide that binds tightly to hydroxyapatite and dental surfaces, suggesting a possible function at tooth surfaces. Holbrook and Molan (1975) found a histidine-rich peptide in parotid saliva that was active in enhancing glycolytic activity of salivary microorganisms. Histidine-rich polypeptides isolated from human parotid saliva show growth-inhibitory and bactericidal effects on *Streptococcus mutans* (MacKay *et al.*, 1984*b*) as well as fungistatic and fungicidal activity against *Candida albicans* (Pollock *et al.*, 1984).

Peters and Azen (1977) purified and partially characterized the Pb proteins. The apparent molecular weights range between 5800 and 7200 and the proteins are extremely basic (45% of the basic residues representing histidine, lysine, and arginine) with isoelectric points above pH 9.5. A model was presented supporting the concept that the polymorphism is due to a combination of allelic differences and posttranslational modifications by deamidation and proteolysis (Peters and Azen, 1977).

Employing an antiserum prepared against human Pb proteins in rabbits, Peters *et al.* (1977) found another protein showing immunological identity to Pb proteins by double diffusion and immunoelectrophoretic analysis. This protein, termed the PPb (post-Pb protein), is similar in molecular weight to the largest protein (e) of the Pb protein series. From the amino acid analysis, the PPb protein resembles the Pb protein; however, from the amino acid sequence analysis, the PPb protein is different and not a precursor of Pb proteins. Thus, it seems likely that the PPb protein is determined by a genetic locus that is distinct from that determining the Pb proteins.

In a comparative study of parotid saliva from anthropoid primates, Azen *et al.* (1978) detailed the evolution of the biochemically and immunologically related Pb and PPb proteins. Immunoelectrophoretic and electrophoretic comparisons suggest that the PPb protein may have evolved in hominoids relatively recently after divergence from the cercopithecoids, but prior to the hylobatid-pongid/hominid divergence. Thus, the *PPb* gene may have evolved from the *Pb* gene by a process of gene duplication.

Other Polymorphisms in Human Saliva

In most of the previously described studies, parotid saliva was used, since it can be obtained almost sterile and uncontaminated by other oral secretions that may lead to variable composition. Also, both Pb and Pr proteins may be altered in whole saliva, probably because of enzymatic degradation or complexing (Oppenheim *et al.*, 1971; Azen, 1973; Friedman *et al.*, 1975). In contrast, the following polymorphisms were detected in whole human saliva. Balakrishnan and Ashton (1974) found polymorphism of a pair of proteins that was detected in alkaline polyacrylamide gels stained with Coomassie brilliant blue. From the genetic analysis, the polymorphism is controlled by two loci, Sal_I and Sal_{II}, each with a dominant and a recessive gene. From the results of electrophoretic comparisons (Azen, 1978a), the Sal proteins may be in the *Pr* system, but the genetic analysis seems inconsistent with this interpretation. The reasons for this inconsistency remain undetermined, but perhaps the use of parotid saliva by Azen and Oppenheim (1973) and Azen and Denniston (1974) versus the use of whole saliva by Balakrishnan and Ashton (1974) may account for these differences.

Other polymorphisms have been found among enzymes in whole saliva as determined by isozyme analysis in polyacrylamide gels. These enzymes include carboxylesterase, glucose-6-phosphate dehydrogenase, and acid phosphatase. Carboxylesterase variants are controlled by an autosomal locus with two codominant alleles, Set_1^F and Set_1^S (Tan, 1976). Glucose-6-phosphate dehydrogenase variants are controlled by an autosomal locus with two alleles, Sgd^1 and Sgd^2 (Tan and Ashton, 1976a). Finally, acid phosphatase variants are the products of two loci, Sap_A with three alleles and Sap_B with two alleles; one of the alleles at each locus is a "null" (Tan and Ashton, 1976b).

MOLECULAR GENETIC STUDIES

The Proline-Rich Protein (PRP) Gene Family

As described previously, protein polymorphism studies have suggested at least 13 genetic loci in the human salivary PRP system, but at the DNA level it is less complex. From the DNA studies, six loci in this gene family control the synthesis of PRPs. The protein complexities arise because each gene is capable of producing more than one PRP. First, each gene product (precursor protein) can generate multiple PRPs by various posttranslational cleavages on the carboxylic side of specific arginine residues. Second, at least with one gene, differential RNA splicing can occur to give multiple transcripts with different lengths. Third, multiple alleles are found at each locus.

In the following sections we will focus on DNA studies that show how a large number of PRPs found in human saliva are generated from a much smaller number of genes.

Six Loci with Two Subfamilies of Genes

In contrast with human saliva, in which PRPs account for about 70% of the protein components, only small amounts of PRPs are found in rat salivary gland (Muenzer *et al.*, 1979). A dramatic increase in the synthesis of PRPs was observed, however, upon treatment of rats with isoproterenol (Ziemer *et al.*, 1982). Using this induction property and the differential hybridization technique, Ziemer *et al.* (1984) successfully isolated cDNAs for rat PRPs from a library prepared from parotid glands of isoproterenol-treated rats. One of the cDNA clones was then used to screen a phage library made from a partial *Eco*RI digest of total human DNA (Azen *et al.*, 1984). Two clones, PRP1 and PRP2, hybridized to the rat cDNA probe under moderately stringent conditions and contained related but not identical DNAs. Both contained regions consisting of nearly identical, tandemly repeated sequences, each able to code for about 21 amino acids and homologous to the repeated amino acid units found in human PRPs by protein sequencing (Wong and Bennick, 1980; Kauffman *et al.*, 1982; Shimomura *et al.*, 1983). This demonstrated that these clones contain members of the PRP gene family.

A DNA probe, *Hinf*I 980, mainly composed of repeats of the gene, was prepared from the PRP1 clone and used to isolate cDNA clones for human PRPs from a cDNA library made from the total poly A + RNA of a single human parotid gland (Maeda *et al.*, 1985). We found that the cDNA clones coding for human PRPs fall into two groups: one group hybridized strongly to the probe even after a stringent wash, and the other group no longer gave strong signals after a stringent wash. By sequencing, it was found that cDNAs of the two groups differ slightly in the structure of the repetitive region. The cDNAs of the first group have repeated nucleotide sequences homologous to those in the clones PRP1 and PRP2. Since the sites for the restriction enzyme *Bst*N1 occur in these repeated regions approximately every 63 bases, they are named *Bst*N1 repeats. The cDNA clones in the second group have, on the other hand, a repeating unit in which a site for the restriction enzyme *Hae*III is present. These repeats are called *Hae*III repeats. The consensus nucleotide and decoded amino acid sequences of *Hae*III and *Bst*N1 type repeats are given in Fig. 1.

This division into two subfamilies is illustrated by the genomic Southern blot shown in Fig. 2. A probe containing *Hae*III-type repeats and one containing *Bst*N1-type repeats both hybridize to the same six *Eco*RI fragments under nonstringent conditions, but after washing under stringent conditions, two fragments remain strongly hybridized to the probe with *Hae*III-type repeats and four remain hybridized to the probe having *Bst*N1-type repeats. Further studies have shown that each of the six fragments detected by DNA hybridization contains only one PRP gene; therefore, these DNA studies suggest that there are six loci coding for PRPs, two of the *Hae*III type (*PRH1, PRH2*) and four of the *Bst*N1 type (*PRB1, PRB2, PRB3, and PRB4*).

The discrepancy between the number of genetic loci postulated by the protein data (at least 13) versus the DNA studies was partly solved by the reexamination of the pattern of inheritance of the PRPs. Maeda (1985) noted that there are no individuals having all three, nor lacking all three, acidic proteins Db, Pa, and PIF, which were postulated to be coded by three discrete loci. It was also noted that the gene frequencies of Pa^+, Db^+, and PIF^+ add to about 1.0 in different racial groups. Based on these observations, it was hypothesized that the three acidic PRPs (Db, Pa, and PIF) are coded by three alleles at a single locus rather than by three discrete loci,

```
              P   P   Q   G   K   P   Q   G   P   P   Q   Q   Q   G   G   H   Q   Q   G   P   P   P
HaeIII  CCTCCTCAAGGAAAGCCACAAGGACCACCCCCAACAGGGAGGCCATCAGCAGCAAGGACCTCCCCCA
               *                                                        *   * **    **** **

BstNI   CCTCCTCCAGGAAAGCCACAAGGACCACCCCCAACAGGAGGCAACAAGCCCCAAGGTCCCCCCA
              P   P   P   G   K   P   Q   G   P   P   Q   Q   Q   G   G   N   K   P   Q   G   P   P   P
```

Fig. 1. Comparison of the consensus nucleotide and amino acid sequence of the repetitive unit of the HaeIII-type and BstN1-type PRP genes. Differences of nucleotides between HaeIII-type and BstN1-type repeats are shown with asterisks. The recognition sites for HaeIII and BstN1 restriction enzymes are underlined.

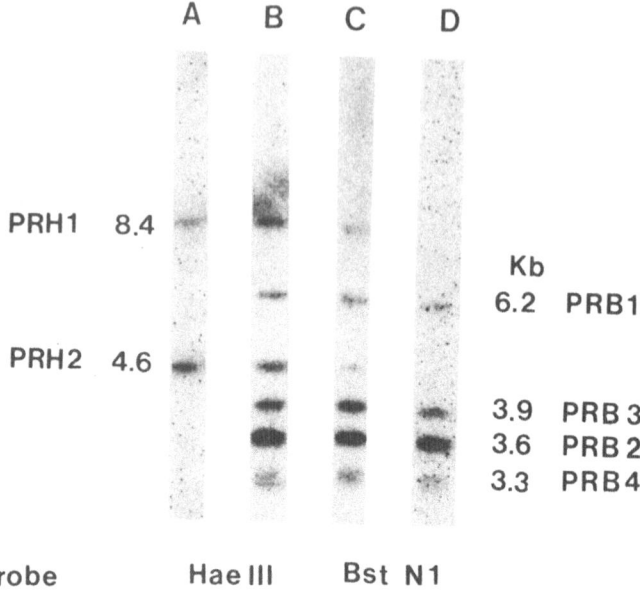

Fig. 2. Southern blot hybridization of *Eco*RI digests of human DNA. The filter was hybridized to a ^{32}P-labeled probe containing *Hae*III-type repeats and washed under nonstringent conditions (lane B), and further washed under more stringent conditions (lane A). Two hybridizing fragments of 8.4 and 4.6 kb remain, and these correspond to *PRH1* and *PRH2*, respectively. When the same filter was rehybridized to a probe containing *Bst*N1-type repeats and washed under nonstringent conditions (lane C), the same six hybridizing bands as in lane B were seen. Further wash of the filter under more stringent conditions (lane D) reveals four hybridizing bands of 6.2, 3.9, 3.6, and 3.3 kb corresponding to *PRB1*, *PRB3*, *PRB2*, and *PRB4*, respectively.

each having a null allele. This hypothesis was proved correct by the DNA study as described below (Azen *et al.*, 1987).

Two *Hae*III-Type Genes Code for Acidic PRPs

To understand fully the complexity of the PRP system, it is necessary to identify all of the genes and their products. We approached this goal by studying structures of *Hae*III-type PRP transcripts and their genes from a single individual whose PRP salivary phenotypes were known.

The nucleotide sequences of cDNA clones with *Hae*III repeats showed that they code for the precursors of acidic PRPs. Figure 3 illustrates the cDNA clone (cP2) of a transcript from the gene at the *PRH1* locus (*PRH1*[4] allele), which codes for an acidic PRP, PIF. A precursor protein coded by the gene is composed of four domains. The secretory signal sequence (S) is composed of 16 predominantly hydrophobic amino acids. The N-terminal region, which is rich in acidic and hydrophobic residues, is divided into two regions: N1 is a region of 17 amino acids and is followed by N2, a region of 36 amino acids. The region (H) consists of 21 amino acid repeats and is rich in proline (there are five repeats in cP2). The small C-terminal region consists of five residues. This overall structure is common to all the transcripts in the PRP genes, except that the N2 region is unique to the *Hae*III-type genes, and there is no counterpart in the *Bst*N1-type genes. The decoded amino acid sequence of the PIF protein is identical (except for one difference) to the amino acid sequence of an acidic PRP, protein C, determined by Wong and Bennick (1980). An aspartic acid occurs at position 50 in PIF instead of asparagine in protein C. Wong and Bennick (1980) have shown that the amino acid sequence of their protein A is identical to the first N-terminal 106 residues of protein C, which is 150 residues in length. The salivary proteinase kallikrein cleaves protein C on the carboxyl side of Arg-106 (Wong *et al.*, 1983) to give protein A plus a C-terminal peptide of 44 amino acids. Isemura *et al.* (1980) identified in saliva a basic PRP peptide, P-C, which is identical in sequence to the 44 C-terminal residues of protein C. Since we did not find *Hae*III-type cDNAs that are missing the C-terminal 44 residues, we conclude that the double-banded patterns of acidic PRPs, such as PIF-fast and PIF-slow proteins, are generated by posttranslational cleavages of the precursor proteins. Therefore, the transcript corresponding to cP2 can generate three proteins, including PIF-slow, PIF-fast, and the P-C peptide.

The transcript for the PIF protein is coded by the *PRH1* locus, whose organization is shown in Fig. 3 as determined by Kim and Maeda (1986). The gene is approximately 3.5 kb in length and contains four exons. The first exon codes for the signal peptide (S) and a part of the first N-terminal region (N1). The second exon codes for the next 12 residues of the N1 region. Exon 3 encodes the N2

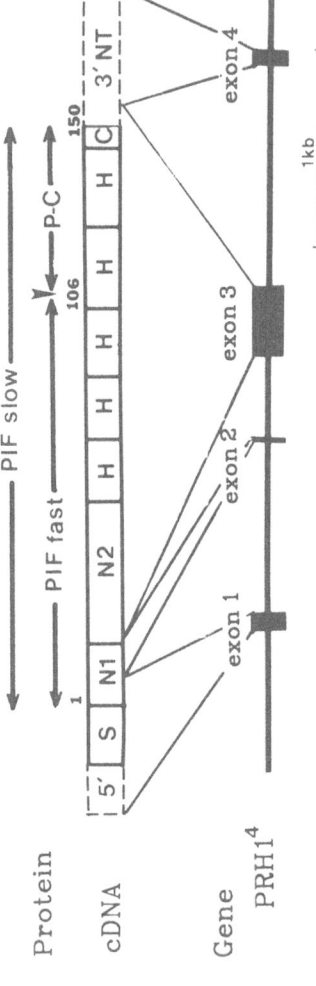

Fig. 3. Structures of a *Hae*III-type gene *PRH1*[4], its transcript, and protein products. The gene spans about 3.5 kb of DNA and contains four exons as shown by black bars. The transcript, analyzed as a cDNA, is about 670 bp long, and has five *Hae*III-type repeating units (H). The precursor protein decoded from the nucleotide sequence of the cDNA has a signal peptide (S), N-terminal regions (N1 and N2), *Hae*III-type repeats (H), and a C-terminal region (C). The mature protein, PIF slow, contains 150 amino acid residues. Partial cleavage can occur at the carboxyl side of Arg-106 (indicated by an arrowhead), generating the PIF-fast peptide of 106 amino acids and the P-C peptide of 44 amino acids.

region, the proline-rich tandem repeats (H), and the C-terminal region (C). Exon 4 codes for the 3' nontranslated part of the message. This organization is common to all of the PRP genes.

Two other alleles at the *PRH1* locus were also cloned and their nucleotide sequences were determined (Azen *et al.*, 1987). This was performed using the genomic DNA of two individuals, one with the protein phenotype Db+, Pa−, and PIF− and the other with the phenotype Db−, Pa+, and PIF−. The *PRH1*[1] allele codes for a precursor of the Db protein, which can be processed to Db slow, Db fast, and the P-C peptide. The nucleotide sequence of the *PRH1*[1] allele differs from that of the *PRH1*[4] allele (coding for PIF) by having eight nucleotide substitutions and six *Hae*III-type repeats instead of five. The extra repeat of the *PRH1*[1] allele is identical to the 3' half of the first and the 5' half of the second repeat of the *PRH1*[4] allele. This result suggests that the extra repeat in *PRH1*[1] has been generated by homologous recombination within the first and second repeat or is the result of slippage during replication of DNA. One nucleotide substitution in exon 3 leads to an amino acid replacement at position 26 (leucine in Db instead of isoleucine in PIF).

The *PRH1*[2] allele codes for a precursor of the Pa protein. The Pa protein is twice as large as the PIF-slow protein, because it forms a dimer with an S–S bond. The Pa protein is also the only acidic PRP that does not show the double-banded phenotype. From the nucleotide sequence, the *PRH1*[2] allele has five *Hae*III-type repeats and three nucleotide substitutions that are different from the eight found in comparing *PRH1*[1] with *PRH1*[4] alleles. One of these substitutions occurs in the third exon and replaces Arg-103 in the PIF and in Db proteins with Cys-103 in the Pa protein. This cysteine residue is involved in the disulfide bonding and structurally interferes with the proteolytic cleavage at Arg-106 in the Pa protein, and this accounts for the single-banded electrophoretic pattern of the Pa protein.

The second *Hae*III-type locus, *PRH2*, codes for precursors of the Pr proteins. There are two common alleles, *PRH2*[1] and *PRH2*[2], which code for Pr-1 and Pr-2, respectively. The amino acid sequence of the Pr-1 protein, predicted from the nucleotide sequence of the cDNA (cP1), differs from that of the PIF protein at two positions:

aspartic acid occurs at position 4 of Pr-1 instead of asparagine in PIF, and asparagine occurs at position 50 of Pr-1 instead of aspartic acid in PIF. At the nucleotide level, the two *Hae*III-type genes (*PRH1*[4] and *PRH2*[1]) differ from each other by an average of 8.7% (Kim and Maeda, 1986). The sequences of exon 3, which contains the *Hae*III-type repeats of the genes, differ by only 0.2%, while those of IVS 3 differ by about 15%. Because of this uneven distribution of sequence differences, these genes have evolved not only by duplication and divergence events, but also by recombinational events between genes within the family.

The Genes in the BstN1 Subfamily Code for Multiple Basic and Glycosylated PRPs

From the nucleotide sequences of the cDNA clones with *Bst*N1-type repeats, Maeda *et al.* (1985) showed that they code for precursor proteins that have a signal peptide (S), an N-terminal region (N1), a repetitive region (B), and a C-terminal region (C), each homologous to the corresponding region in precursors coded by the *Hae*III-type genes. However, in contrast to *Hae*III-type cDNAs, there is no N2 region in the *Bst*N1-type precursor.

The *Bst*N1-type cDNA clone cP3 derived from the *PRB1* locus is shown in Fig. 4. The *Bst*N1-type repeats can be subdivided into B1, B2, and B3 types and the "B1–B2–B3" unit occurs four times in cP3. At the end of each B3 repeat, there is a codon for an arginine residue, except for the third B3 repeat, in which there is a codon for glutamine. The "B1–B2–B3" unit codes for 61 amino acids, and the sequence is very similar, although not identical, to the amino acid sequences of basic PRPs so far sequenced. From this result, a single transcript of a *Bst*N1-type gene can code for a precursor protein that can be cleaved posttranslationally to generate multiple products. Therefore, from the mRNA corresponding to the cP3 clone, at least four peptides can be generated, and, if the cleavage at each Arg residue is not complete (as in the case of acidic PRPs), up to ten PRP peptides are expected.

Another important mechanism for generating multiple PRPs

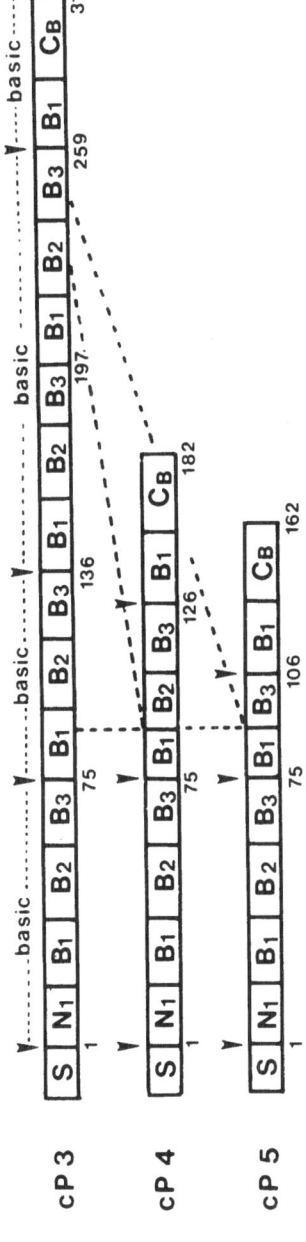

Fig. 4.   Summary of the PRP precursor protein structure of a *Bst*N1-type gene. The structures of proteins decoded from the nucleotide sequence of cDNAs cP3, cP4, and cP5 are identical, except that cP4 and cP5 are missing middle parts of cP3 due to the differential splicing of mRNA. The precursor proteins have signal peptides (S), N-terminal regions (N1), *Bst*N1-type repeats (subtypes are designated as B_1, B_2, and B_3), and C-terminal regions (C_B). Basic peptides are generated after posttranslational cleavage at sites indicated by arrowheads.

from a single gene is by differential RNA splicing from the mRNA of a single gene, which generates multiple mRNAs of different lengths (Maeda *et al.*, 1985). Two cDNA clones (cP4 and cP5) were missing 399 and 459 bp, respectively, from the repetitive region of cP3. The sequences at these deletion endpoints are homologous to the consensus sequence of RNA splicing donor and acceptor sites, suggesting that all three cDNAs are derived from transcripts of a single gene via differential RNA splicing. Because of its repeated structure, the cP3 clone carries two possible donor sites and eight possible acceptor sites in the sequence. We do not know whether or not all the possible sites are used. As illustrated in Fig. 4, these transcripts of different lengths contribute to the number of PRP peptides that can be generated from a gene at the *PRB1* locus.

The second *Bst*N1-type locus, *PRB2*, is highly homologous to *PRB1*, judging from the partial nucleotide sequence analysis of the *PRB2* and *PRB1* clones [formerly termed *PRP2* and *PRP1*, respectively (Azen *et al.*, 1984)]. The cDNA clone cP7 corresponds to the transcript of *PRB2* and is a partial cDNA that contains only the 3' part of the gene. Although retaining the "B1–B2–B3" unit structure, cP7 differs from cP3 by having a sugar attachment site "N–X–S" in the decoded sequence of some of the repeats. Posttranslational cleavages will generate various small basic glycopeptides from this gene. Variations in the degree of glycosylation of the basic PRPs have been described by Bennick (1982); thus, some contain no carbohydrate, but others contain 1.7–5.2 sugar residues per 100 amino acids. From partial characterization of the *PRP2* clone (Azen *et al.*, 1984), the gene contains approximately 15 *Bst*N1-type repeats.

Another type of glycosylated PRP is coded by the *Bst*N1-type gene *PRB4*. The cDNA clone cP6, which corresponds to the transcript of *PRB4*, has a fourth variety of *Bst*N1-type repeat, which also has a sugar attachment site in the decoded sequence. After posttranslational cleavage, it can generate a basic glycopeptide of 138 amino acids with six sugar chains and a basic peptide of 70 amino acids, whose amino acid sequence, except for one amino acid difference, corresponds to that of P-D determined by Saitoh *et al.* (1983*c*).

The organization and structure of *PRB4* and *PRB3* (Lyons *et*

Giemsa banding, 9
Glucose-6-phosphate
    dehydrogenase, 53
Glycoprotein metabolism
    disorders listed, 13

Hemophilia, human, 27–59
    A, factor VIII, deficiency, 27–59
    cloning, 28
    DNA, 28, 32
    gene, 28–44
        and DNA polymorphism,
            40–44
        genetics, molecular, 27–59
    mutation, 32–40
        deletion, 33–36
        hot spots, 32, 39, 40
        listed, 32, 35
        nucleotide substitution,
            single, 36–40
    protein sequence, 28–32
    mRNA, 31
    schema of, 29, 31
    B, factor IX, deficiency,
        27–59
    Alabama, 50
    amino acid sequence of
        bovine, 44
    Chapel Hill, 49–50
    characterization, 44–46
    cloning, 44–46
    DNA, 45, 51–52
        polymorphism in gene,
            51–52
    gene, 44–52
    mutation, 46–51
        deletion, 46–49
        DNA polymorphism, 51–52
        of nucleotide, single, 49–51
    nucleotide sequence of gene,
        44
    protein domains of gene, 44,
        45

Hemophilia, human (*cont.*)
    B, factor IX, deficiency (*cont.*)
        mRNA, 45
        is serine protease, 27
        X-chromosome mapping, 53
    factor X, 28
Heart defect, congenital
    and imbalance, chromosomal, 99
HeLa cell
    cDNA clone, pUNC*724*,
        112–118
    on short arm, acrocentric,
        112–118
Hysteroscopy, transcervical, 3

Index, mitotic, 9

Kugelberg–Welander disease, 63

Lesch–Nyhan syndrome, 71
Lipid, neutral, metabolism
    disorders listed, 12

Metabolic disease
    inherited, 10
    listed, 12–14; *see also separate
        diseases*
Methylmalonate metabolism
    disorders listed, 14
Mucopolysaccharide metabolism
    disorders listed, 13
Muscle, skeletal, human
    DNA analysis, 87–88
    protein, 87–89

Nebulin, 89
Nondisjunction in trisomy 21,
    99–140
    and age, maternal, 102–104,
        128–129
    of chromosome 21: *see* Trisomy
        21

Nondisjunction in trisomy (*cont.*)
  and conceptus phenotype, 109–
    110, 131–132
  and couples at high risk, 129
  and crossing-over,
    chromosomal, 106–109,
    130–131
  design, experimental, proposed,
    126–127
  and irradiation, maternal, 105
  origin, parental, 100–102,
    127–128
  phenotype of conceptus, 109–
    110, 131–132
  pilot study of five families,
    123–126
  problems listed, 100

Ornithine transcarbamylase
    deficiency, 73
Ovum, fertilized, 2

Parotid gland basic proteins,
    170–171
  histidine-rich, 170–171
Peroxidase, salivary, 169–170
Plasmid
  and chromosome walking, 113
  pUNC724, 112–118
Pompe disease, 63
Proline-rich protein, salivary, 149,
    150, 156–168
  alleles, multiple, 183–184
  acidic, 156–168, 176–185
  basic, 156, 157, 160, 170–171,
    180–183
  concanavalin A-binding, 167
  double band, 163–164
  genes, 176–185
    cluster, 184–185
    and chromosome
      localization, 184–185
  structure, 178

Proline-rich protein (*cont.*)
  genetics, molecular, 172–176
  genes, 173–176
  loci, 173–176
  glycoprotein, major parotid,
    165–166
  glycosylated, 156, 157, 180–183
  loci, 173–176, 184
  parotid
    heavy protein, 166
    isoelectric focusing variant,
      164
    middle band protein
      fast, 164–165
      slow, 165
    size variant, 161
  Pc protein, 168
  Pe protein, 167–168
  polymorphism, 156–168
  Po protein, 168
Propionate metabolism
  disorders listed, 14
Protein, salivary, human 141–199
  listed, 143–153
  polymorphism, 142–172
  proline-rich: *see* Proline-rich
    protein
  see also Nebulin, B_{12}-binding
    protein

Retardation, mental
  and imbalance chromosomal, 99
  in dystrophy, muscular, 87
R-protein, 155

Saliva, human, 141–199; *see also*
    Proline-rich protein,
    Protein, salivary
Sphingolipid metabolism
  disorders listed, 12
Statherin, 185–187
  amino acid composition, 185
  chromosome localization, 186
Stefin, 190

Tannin, 156–157
Transabdominal technique, 7–8
Transcervical technique, 3–8
  aspiration by catheter, 4–6
  biopsy forceps, 6–7
  endoscopy, 6
  hysteroscopy, 3
  infection due to, 8
Transcobalamin II of plasma, 155
Trisomy 21, 99–140
  and age, maternal, 102–104
  and conceptus phenotype,
    109–110
  couples identified for risk,
    104–106
  and origin, parental, 100–102,
    109–110
    nondisjunction, parental,
      100–102
  and phenotype of conceptus,
    109–110
  and polymorphism, cytogenetic,
    101
Trophoblast
  development, early, 2–3
  differentiation, 2

Ultrasound for guidance, 5

Urea cycle constituent
  disorders listed, 13

Villus, chorionic
  sampling during first trimester,
    1–25
    analysis, metabolic, 10–15
    chromosome analysis, 8–10
    contraindication for, 17
    diagnosis, metabolic, 10–15
      pitfalls, 14–15
    disorders, metabolic, listed,
      12–14
    DNA analysis, 4, 15–16
      disorders listed, 16
    history, 3–4
    karyotype analysis, 8–9
    mosaicism, 10
    processing, 8
    safety of, 17–18
      risk of abortion,
        spontaneous, 17–18
    techniques for, 4–8
      transabdominal, 7–8
      transcervical, 4–7
      ultrasound guidance, 5
    see also Trophoblast
von Willebrand factor, 30

X-chromosome mapping, 53–54

al., submitted) suggest that these two loci are very similar in structure and that the gene at *PRB3* also generates heavily glycosylated PRPs. Thus, structurally four *Bst*N1-type genes can be further divided into two subtypes; *PRB1* and *PRB2* form one subtype, and *PRB3* and *PRB4* form a second subtype. Many basic and glycosylated PRP peptides can be generated from these genes.

Multiple Alleles with Different Number of Repeats

The complexity of PRP proteins in saliva also arises because of the existence of common multiple alleles at each of the six PRP loci. As discussed above, there are three common alleles at the *PRH1* locus, and one of them, *PRH1*[1] (Db), has an extra repeat compared to the other two. Alleles with different numbers of repeats are also commonly found at the four *Bst*N1-type loci. When Southern blots of DNA digests of unrelated individuals are probed with a labeled fragment (*Hinf*I 980) from the repetitive region of PRP 1 (*PRB1*), frequent doublets are seen with typically less than 1 kb difference between the two components of each pair (Azen *et al.*, 1984). These polymorphisms are due to length differences rather than mutations at restriction sites, since digestion of the DNAs with several restriction enzymes reveals a qualitatively similar doublet pattern. Lyons *et al.* (1988*a*) analyzed the alleles of the four *Bst*N1-type loci at the nucleotide sequence level and showed that the length differences were generated by homologous unequal crossing over within the repeats between sister or homologous strands.

Correlations between insertion/deletion RFLPs and PRP protein phenotypes, as well as comparison of nucleotide and decoded amino acid sequences from each of four *Bst*N1-type loci with the available protein sequence data, allowed tentative assignments of the following polymorphic PRPs (Table III): PmF, PmS, and Pe proteins to the *PRB1* locus, the Ps protein to the *PRB2* locus, the G1 protein to the *PRB3* locus, and the Po, Con 1, and Con 2 proteins to the *PRB4* locus (Lyons *et al.*, 1988*b*). The Pc polymorphic protein is probably a proteolytic cleavage product of a PRB locus, but a specific assignment has not yet been made. In several cases, basic

TABLE III. Summary of PRP Genes, Their Alleles and Their Products

Family	Locus	Allele	Product	Size of *Eco*RI genomic fragment (kb)
*Hae*III type	*PRH1*	*PRH1*[1]	Db-slow, Db-fast, P-C	
		PRH1[2]	Pa 1	
		PRH1[3]	Pa 2	8.4
		PRH1[4]	PIF-slow, PIF-fast, P-C	
	PRH2	*PRH2*[1]	Pr 1, Pr 3, P-C	
		PRH2[2]	Pr 2, Pr 4, P-C	4.6
		PRH2[3]	Pr 1', Pr 3-like, P-C-like	
*Bst*N1 type	*PRB1*	Several	DEAEII-2 (Pe), IB-6 (PmS), IB-9 (P-F), P-H	6.2
	PRB2	Several	P-H, Ps	3.6
	PRB3	Several	G1, CDII-f	3.9
	PRB4	Several	P-D (Po), Con 1, Con 2, CDII-g	3.3

PRPs that were previously considered to be products of separate loci are actually proteolytic cleavage products of a large precursor specified by a *Bst*N1-type gene. It is likely that "null" alleles proposed to occur at *Bst*N1-type genes in earlier genetic studies are really productive alleles having alterations at proteolytic cleavage sites in the precursor proteins. The absence of cleavage may lead to longer precursor proteins that could not be resolved electrophoretically (Lyons *et al.*, 1988*b*). In Table III, the PRP loci, their alleles, and possible products are summarized. Assignments of all the PRPs to specific loci await further protein sequence studies and correlations between the variations in the DNA sequences and the phenotypes of the salivary proteins.

Chromosomal Localization of the PRP Gene Cluster

A PRP DNA probe, *Hinf*I 980, was used to analyze segregation of human PRP genes in human–mouse somatic cell hybrids, and the human PRP gene family was localized to chromosome 12 (Azen *et* *al.*, 1985). The same probe was also used by Mamula *et al.* (1985) to localize the PRP gene complex to a single band 12p13.2 by *in situ* hybridization. Since the probe detects frequent DNA length polymorphisms, it is very useful for genetic linkage studies with other chromosome 12 markers. Thus, O'Connell *et al.* (1987) localized the PRP gene cluster between *KRAS2* and *VWF*. The most likely order and orientation are *-KRAS2-[PRB2-PRB1-PRB(3,4)]-VWF*-12pter. From linkage analysis of proline-rich protein polymorphisms, Goodman *et al.* (1985) reported approximately 15% recombination across the PRP loci. O'Connell *et al.* (1987) did two-point analyses with RFLP markers to determine estimates of recombination among the four PRB loci. They estimated about 3% recombination across the PRB loci. The reason for the discrepancy in recombination estimates is not clear.

H.-S. Kim, O. Smithies, and N. Maeda (in preparation) independently obtained the physical map of the gene cluster by combination of the linking library and pulsed field gel electrophoresis. Their result shows that the PRP gene cluster spans about 700 kb of DNA and the genes are most likely arranged in the order and distance of *PRB2*-(60 kb)-*PRB1*-(70 kb)-*PRB4*-(190 kb)-*PRH2*-(160 kb)-*PRB3*-(190 kb)-*PRH1*. This physical arrangement of the genes, together with their structural relatedness, indicates that the PRP gene family has expanded to the current six members via a series of homologous unequal crossover events.

Statherin

Statherin plays an important role in maintaining oral health, since, together with anionic PRPs, it binds calcium, inhibits crystal growth, and exhibits a high affinity for hydroxyapatite (Bennick, 1982). Statherin is a small-molecular weight (5380), acidic (pI 4.2), human salivary protein that is rich in tyrosine, proline, and glutamine. Its complete amino acid sequence has been determined (Schlesinger and Hay, 1977). Statherin and acidic PRPs maintain a supersaturated state with respect to calcium phosphate salts and prevent the accumulation of harmful deposits on tooth surfaces or in salivary glands (Hay *et al.*, 1984). This activity also protects the teeth by preventing dissolution of dental enamel and permits recalcification of early carious lesions. The concentration of statherin in parotid saliva varies tenfold between individuals and ranges from 3.0 to >27.3 μM (Hay *et al.*, 1984). Based on the known amino acid sequence of statherin (Schlesinger and Hay, 1977), Sabatini *et al.* (1987) constructed two mixed synthetic oligonucleotide probes that were used to isolate a statherin cDNA clone from a human parotid gland cDNA library. The nucleotide sequence of the cDNA insert (672 bp) and its decoded amino acid sequence are compatible with the known 43-amino acid sequence of statherin (Schlesinger and Hay, 1977). The primary translation product includes a 19-amino acid secretory signal peptide. Analysis of the parotid gland RNA reveals a major hybridizing RNA species approximately 640 nucleotides in length. Thus, the cDNA clone contains a full- or nearly full-length cDNA copy of statherin mRNA.

The number of copies of statherin DNA present in the human genome was estimated at one copy per haploid genome by comparing the intensity of hybridization of a statherin gene fragment in genomic DNA with varying known amounts of the same cloned fragment.

The statherin gene was localized to the chromosome 4q11–13 region by hybridizing a statherin gene fragment to endonuclease-digested DNAs of human–Chinese hamster somatic cell hybrids, one of which contained only human chromosome 4 and others that contained intact or various deletions of chromosome 4. Several markers are known to be in the same region as statherin (McKusick, 1986). These markers include: peptidase S (PEPS), metallothionein 2-processed pseudogene (MT2P1), α-fetoprotein (AFP), albumin (ALB), group-specific component (GC), and dentinogenesis imperfecta (DGI1). Hereditary persistence of α-fetoprotein (HPAFP) and juvenile periodontitis (JP) have also been provisionally localized to this region of chromosome 4. It is interesting that statherin maps in the same region as two dental disorders, DGI1 and JP. The disorder DGI1 is an autosomal dominant mutation of dental tissue protein matrix dentin, with clinically normal or hypoplastic enamel formation. Since tooth defects are apparent prior to tooth eruption, saliva protein may not play a role in this process; however, the possibility that statherin may be expressed in the tooth bud has not yet been investigated. Further genetic and cytogenetic mapping of the statherin gene will be necessary in order to investigate a possible linkage with these disorders.

Amylase Gene Family

Alpha-amylase catalyses the digestion of starch and glycogen. The structure and evolution of the amylase gene family have recently been reviewed (Meisler and Gumucio, 1986). In mammals, the clustered amylase gene family contains two types of genes, which are expressed in either pancreas or salivary gland. There is close linkage of human amylase genes on chromosome 1 as determined by pedigree analysis (Merritt and Karn, 1977). More recently, Zabel et al. (1983), using a human amylase gene probe, assigned the amylase gene to lp21 by in situ hybridization. Tricoli and Shows (1984) hybridized a human amylase DNA probe to endonuclease-digested DNAs of somatic cell hybrids and mapped amylase genes to the 1p21–1p22.1 region. Nakamura et al. (1984) determined the nucleotide sequences of cloned human salivary and pancreatic α-amylase cDNAs, including all of the amino acid-coding regions. Subsequently, Nishide et al. (1986a) corrected some errors in the sequences of the cDNAs for the human salivary and pancreatic α-amylases as published by Nakamura et al. (1984). The nucleotide sequences of the two cDNAs are 98% homologous in the coding region, and the derived amino acid sequences are 97% homologous. Nakamura et al. (1984) suggested the possibility of gene conversion between human salivary and pancreatic α-amylase genes after comparing predicted amino acid sequences of human and mouse α-amylases. Wise et al. (1984) also isolated a cDNA sequence for human pancreatic amylase.

Nishide et al. (1986b) determined the primary structure of a human salivary α-amylase gene by using a human salivary α-amylase cDNA probe to screen a genomic library. From restriction mapping and DNA sequencing, the gene is approximately 10 kb long, with 11 exons and 10 introns. The 5' flanking sequence surrounding the

CAT box is highly homologous with that of the mouse salivary α-amylase gene, suggesting a role in tissue-specific expression in the salivary gland.

Gumucio *et al.* (1988) isolated and characterized cosmid clones containing 250 kb of genomic DNA from the human amylase gene cluster. To do this, they screened a cosmid library with a mixture of salivary and pancreatic amylase cDNAs from A/J mice. They identified, by sequence comparison with cDNAs, three salivary amylase genes, two pancreatic amylase genes, and two truncated pseudogenes. An intergenic distance of 17–24 kb separated genes that were linked by chromosomal walking. The three human salivary amylase genes must be very similar, since *Eco*RI, *Hind*III, and *Bam*HI restriction maps are identical throughout a 27-kb region, and there is sequence identity among 950 nucleotides that were compared. However, the two human pancreatic amylase genes differ in their restriction maps, and the 5′ flanking sequences are divergent. Gumucio *et al.* (1985) used a fragment from the salivary amylase gene to probe Southern blots of endonuclease-digested genomic DNAs and found two RFLPs with *Pst*I ($p = 0.85$, $q = 0.15$) and *Taq*I ($p = 0.97$, $q = 0.03$). Ishizaki *et al.* (1985), using a human salivary amylase cDNA, detected an RFLP after double digestion of genomic DNA with *Pst*I and *Bam*HI. In Japanese, the frequencies of the two alleles are 0.55 and 0.45.

The 5′ flanking regions of the human genes were compared to those of the mouse in order to determine elements involved in tissue-specific expression and hormonal regulation. The 5′ flanking sequences of the human and murine pancreatic genes are highly homologous between nucleotides − 175 and the cap site. Two sequence elements that may influence pancreas-specific expression were found in this region, as well as glucocorticoid regulatory elements and core enhancer sequences. In contrast, the homology of the 5′ flanking region of the human and mouse salivary amylase genes is limited to several short sequences with different orientations and positions in the two species. Some of these sequence elements are found in other genes that are expressed in the parotid gland. The promoter region of the human salivary amylase gene is strikingly different from that of the rodent, where transcription can be initiated from two alternative promoters, the parotid-specific promoter and the liver promoter (Young *et al.*, 1981). The distance between the parotid specific nontranslated exon and exon a is 7.6 kb in the mouse, but only 0.35 kb in the human, suggesting that a portion of the region may have been deleted during evolution. The promoter that is active in rodent liver is not detectable within the 0.35-kb intron of the human salivary amylase gene, and the gene is not transcribed in the human liver.

Cystatin Gene Family

Human saliva contains multiple forms of cysteine-proteinase inhibitors (Minakata and Asano, 1984). They have different isoelectric points of about 4.5, 6.8, and 8.2 and a molecular weight of about 13,000. Isemura *et al.* (1984) purified one of these inhibitors, an acidic protein termed cystatin S, and determined its amino acid sequence. Cystatin S inhibits papain and ficin strongly, and stem bromelin and bovine cathepsin C partially. Two more inhibitors, cystatin SN, with a neutral pI (Isemura *et al.*, 1986*a*), and cystatin SA, with an acidic pI (Isemura *et al.*, 1986*b*), have subsequently been isolated and characterized. In addition, proteins that have shorter N-terminal regions but are otherwise identical to cystatin S, SN, or SA were isolated from saliva. It is suggested that these shorter proteins are degraded forms that are generated by amino peptidase-like activities in saliva, and that the N-terminal portion of the molecule may play a part in the inhibitory activity (Isemura *et al.*, 1986*c*).

Salivary type cystatins were also found in tears, urine, and seminal plasma (Abrahamson *et al.*, 1986). Their amino acid sequences share a high degree of homology with cystatin C (γ trace) (Grubb and Löfberg, 1982; Brizn *et al.*, 1984), which is abundant in human cerebrospinal fluid, seminal plasma, and milk. A variant of cystatin C is a major component of the proteins of the amyloid fibrils in patients with hereditary cerebral hemorrhage with amyloidosis of the Icelandic type (Ghiso *et al.*, 1986).

Saitoh *et al.* (1987) prepared synthetic oligonucleotides corresponding to a part of the amino acid sequence of cystatin S and used them as a probe to screen a cDNA library made from mRNA of a human submandibular gland. One of the clones that contains the C-terminal part of the salivary cystatin gene was then used to isolate three cystatin family genes. Two of the genes, *CST1* and *CST2*, code, respectively, for cystatin SN and SA, and the third gene, *CSTP1*, is a pseudogene. The genes span approximately 3.5 kb of DNA and are composed of three exons. The *CSTP1* gene is a pseudogene, because there are several inactivating mutations in its DNA sequence: the lack of a typical ATA box; the absence of an initiation codon at the corresponding position of initiation codons of *CST1* and *CST2*; the presence of a premature termination codon in the first exon; and the presence of a frameshift deletion mutation in the second exon.

Genomic Southern blots probed with a fragment containing exon 1 and a part of intron 1 from the *CST1* gene indicate that the human salivary cystatin genes are members of a multigene family, probably consisting of seven genes. In addition to the three genes that were characterized, one other member of the same family is expected to code for another salivary protein, cystatin S. It is also highly probable that loci corresponding to the nonsalivary proteins cystatin C and the amyloid fibril protein are included in this seven-member multigene family.

In contrast to the cystatin family of extracellular cysteine-proteinase inhibitors having two disulfide bonds, the stefin family of intracellular inhibitors lacks disulfide bonds. Although representative amino acid sequences of the two families are distinctly different, they are related and of similar low molecular weight (about 10,000–14,000). The cysteine-proteinase inhibitors with high molecular weight (50,000–58,000) are members of the kininogen family. Three cystatinlike domains have been identified in the human kininogen heavy chain (Kitamura *et al.*, 1985; Salvesen *et al.*, 1986; Müller-Esterl *et al.*, 1986) and each domain is composed of three exons. The finding that three exons in the cystatin genes are approximately equal in length to the equivalent exons in the kininogen domains is strong evidence that all the cysteine-proteinase inhibitors form a superfamily of genes derived from a common ancestor.

ACKNOWLEDGMENTS.   Some of the authors' work cited in this review was supported by National Institutes of Health grants DEO 3658-22 and GM20069. This paper is No. 2942 from the Laboratory of Genetics. We thank M. Meisler and colleagues for sending us their manuscript before publication. We also thank L. Sabatini, H.-S. Kim, E. Saitoh, and K. Lyons in our laboratory for permitting us to quote their data prior to publication. Many of the DNA studies described in this review are the result of their hard work. We also acknowledge the support and encouragement of O. Smithies in carrying out molecular analysis of human PRP genes.

REFERENCES

Abrahamson, M., Barrett, A. J., Salvesen, G., and Grubb, A., 1986, Isolation of six proteinase inhibitors from human urine, *J. Biol. Chem.* **261**:11282–11289.

Allen, R. H., 1975, Human vitamin B_{12} transport proteins, in: *Progress in Hematology*, Vol. 9 (E. B., Brown, ed.), pp. 57–84, Grune and Stratton, New York.

Anderson, L. C., and Mandel, I. D., 1982, Salivary protein polymorphisms in caries-resistant adults, *J. Dent. Res.* **61**:1167–1168.

Anderson, L. C., Kauffman, D. L., and Keller, P. J., 1982a, Identification of Pm and PmS human parotid salivary proteins as basic proline-rich proteins, *Biochem. Genet.* **20**:1131–1137.

Anderson, L. C., Lamberts, B. L., and Bruton, W. F. J., 1982b, Salivary protein polymorphisms in caries-free and caries-active adults, *J. Dent. Res.* **61**:393–396.

Azen, E. A., 1972, Genetic polymorphism of basic proteins from parotid saliva, *Science* **176**:673–674.

Azen, E. A., 1973, Properties of salivary basic proteins showing polymorphism, *Biochem. Genet.* **9**:69–86.

Azen, E. A., 1977, Salivary peroxidase (SAPX): Genetic modification and relationship to the proline-rich (Pr) and acidic (Pa) proteins, *Biochem. Genet.* **15**:9–29.

Azen, E. A., 1978a, Genetic protein polymorphisms in human saliva: An interpretive review, *Biochem. Genet.* **16**:79–99.

Azen, E. A., 1978b, Phosphorylation of proline-rich, double band, acidic and post-Pb proteins of human saliva, *Arch. Oral Biol.* **23**:1173–1176.

Azen, E. A., 1978c, Salivary peroxidase activity and thiocyanate concentration in human subjects with genetic variants of salivary peroxidase, *Arch. Oral Biol.* **23**:801–805.

Azen, E. A., 1985, Genetic variation of salivary peroxidase, in: *The Lactoperoxidase System, Chemistry and Biologic Significance* (K. M. Pruitt and J. O. Tenovuo, eds.), pp. 89–97, Marcel Dekker, New York.

Azen, E. A., 1988, Genetic protein polymorphisms of human saliva in: *Clinical Chemistry of Human Saliva* (J. Tenovuo, ed.), CRC Press, Boca Raton, Florida (in press).

Azen, E. A., and Denniston, C. L., 1974, Genetic polymorphism of human salivary proline-rich proteins: Further genetic analysis, *Biochem. Genet.* **12**:109–120.

Azen, E. A., and Denniston, C., 1979, Genetic polymorphism of vitamin B_{12} binding (R) proteins of human saliva detected by isoelectric focusing, *Biochem. Genet.* **17**:909–920.

Azen, E. A., and Denniston, C., 1980, Polymorphism of Ps (parotid size variant) and detection of a protein (PmS) related to the Pm (parotid middle band) system with genetic linkage of *Ps* and *Pm* to *Gl, Db* and *Pr* genetic determinants, *Biochem. Genet.* **18**:483–501.

Azen, E. A., and Denniston, C., 1981, Genetic polymorphism of PIF (parotid isoelectric focusing variant) proteins with linkage to the PPP (parotid proline-rich protein) gene complex, *Biochem. Genet.* **19**:475–485.

Azen, E. A., and Oppenheim, F. G., 1973, Genetic polymorphism of proline-rich human salivary proteins, *Science* **180**:1067–1069.

Azen, E. A., and Yu, P. L., 1984a, Genetic polymorphism of Con 1 and Con 2 salivary proteins detected by immunologic and concanavalin A reactions on nitrocellulose with linkage of Con 1 and Con 2 genes to the SPC (salivary protein gene complex), *Biochem. Genet.* **22**:1–19.

Azen, E. A., and Yu, P. L., 1984b, Genetic polymorphisms of Pe and Po salivary proteins with probable linkage of their genes to the salivary protein gene complex (SPC), *Biochem. Genet.* **22**:1065–1080.

Azen, E. A., Leutenegger, W., and Peters, E. H., 1978, Evolutionary and dietary aspects of salivary basic (Pb) and post Pb (PPb) proteins in anthropoid primates, *Nature* **273**:775–778.

Azen, E. A., Hurley, C. K., and Denniston, C., 1979, Genetic polymorphism of the major parotid salivary glycoprotein (G1) with linkage to the genes for Pr, Db and Pa, *Biochem. Genet.* **17**:257–279.

Azen, E. A., Lyons, K. M., McGonigal, T., Barrett, H. L., Clements, L. S., Maeda, N., Vanin, E. F., Carlson, D. M., and Smithies, O., 1984, Clones from the human gene complex coding for salivary proline-rich proteins, *Proc. Natl. Acad. Sci. USA* **81**:5561–5565.

Azen, E. A., Goodman, P. A., and Lalley, P. A., 1985, Human salivary proline-rich protein genes on chromosomal 12, *Am. J. Hum. Genet.* **37**:418–424.

Azen, E. A., Lush, E. I., and Taylor, B., 1986, Close linkage of mouse genes for salivary proline-rich proteins and taste, *Trends Genet.* **2**:199–200.

Azen, E. A., Kim, H.-S., Goodman, P., Flynn, S., and Maeda, N., 1987, Alleles at the *PRH1* locus coding for the human salivary acidic proline-rich proteins (PRPs) Pa, Db and PIF, *Am. J. Hum. Genet.* **41**:1035–1047.

Balakrishnan, C. R., and Ashton, G. C., 1974, Polymorphism of human salivary proteins, *Am. J. Hum. Genet.* **26**:145–153.

Balekjian, A. Y., and Longton, R. W., 1973, Histones isolated from human parotid fluid, *Biochem. Biophys. Res. Commun.* **50**:676–682.

Baum, B. J., Bird, J. L., Millar, D. B., and Longton, R. W., 1976, Studies on histidine-rich polypeptides from human parotid saliva, *Arch. Biochem. Biophys.* **177**:427–436.

Bennick, A., 1977, Chemical and physical characterization of a phosphoprotein, protein C, from human saliva and comparison with a related protein A, *Biochem. J.* **163**:229–239.

Bennick, A., 1982, Salivary proline-rich proteins, *Mol. Cell Biochem.* **45**:83–99.

Bennick, A., 1987, Structural and genetic aspects of proline-rich proteins, *J. Dent. Res.* **66**:457–461.

Boackle, J., and Suddick, R. P., 1980, Salivary proteins and oral health, in: *The Biologic Basis of Dental Caries* (R. E. Morhart and J. M. Navia, eds.), pp. 113–131, Harper and Row, Hagerstown, Maryland.

Boettcher, B., and de la Lande, F. A., 1969, Electrophoresis of human saliva and identification of inherited variants of amylase isoenzymes, *Aust. J. Exp. Biol. Med. Sci.* **47**:97–103.

Brizn, J., Popovic, T., and Turk, V., 1984, Human cystatin, a new protein inhibitor of cysteine proteinases, *Biochem. Biophys. Res. Commun.* **118**:103–109.

Carmel, R., and Herbert, V., 1969, Deficiency of vitamin B12-binding α-globulin in two brothers, *Blood* **33**:1–12.

Daiger, S. P., Labowe, M. L., Parsons, M., Wang, L., and Cavalli-Sforza, L. L., 1978, Detection of genetic variation with radioactive ligands. III. Genetic polymorphism of transcobalamin II in human plasma, *Am. J. Hum. Genet.* **30**:202–214.

Daniels, T. E., and Newbrun, E., 1966, Measurement of protein and free and bound carbohydrate in human parotid saliva, *Arch. Oral Biol.* **11**:1171–1180.

De Soyza, K., 1978, Polymorphism of human salivary amylase, a preliminary communication, *Hum. Genet.* **45**:189–192.

Eckersall, P. D., and Beeley, J. A., 1981, Genetic analysis of human salivary α-amylase isoenzymes by isoelectric focusing, *Biochem. Genet.* **19**:1055–1062.

Fráter-Schröeder, M., Hitzig, W. H., and Butler, R., 1979, Studies of transcobalamin (TC). I. Detection of TCII isoproteins in human serum, *Blood* **53**:193–203.

Friedman, E. D., Merritt, A. D., and Rivas, M. L., 1975, Genetic studies of human acidic salivary protein (Pa), *Am. J. Hum. Genet.* **27**:292–303.

Ghiso, J., Jensson, O., and Frangione, B., 1986, Amyloid fibrils in hereditary cerebral hemorrhage with amyloidosis of icelandic type is a variant of γ-trace basic protein (cystatin C), *Proc. Natl. Acad. Sci. USA* **83**:2974–2978.

Goodman, P. A., and Karn, R. C., 1983, Human parotid size polymorphism (Ps): Characterization of the two allelic products, Ps 1 and Ps 2 by limited proteolysis, *Biochem. Genet.* **21**:405–416.

Goodman, P. A., Yu, P. L., Azen, E. A., and Karn, R. C., 1985, The human salivary protein complex (SPC): A large block of related genes, *Am. J. Hum. Genet.* **37**:785–797.

Grubb, A., Löfberg, H., 1982, Human γ-trace, a basic microprotein: Amino acid sequence and presence in adenohypophesis, *Proc. Natl. Acad. Sci. USA* **79**:3024–3027.

Gumucio, D. L., Meisler, M. H., and Kidd, J. R., 1985, Detection of two RFLPS near the human salivary amylase gene on the short arm of human chromosome 1, *Am. J. Hum. Genet.* **37**:A155.

Gumucio, D. L., Wiebauer, K., Caldwell, R. M., Samuelson, L. C., and Meisler, M. H., 1988, II. Concerted evolution of the human amylase genes, *Mol. Cell Biol.* **8**:1197–1205.

Hay, D. I., 1975, Fractionation of human parotid salivary proteins and the isolation of a histidine-rich acidic peptide which shows high affinity for hydroxyapatite surfaces, *Arch. Oral Biol.* **20**:553–558.

Hay, D. I., and Oppenheim, F. G., 1974, The isolation from human parotid saliva of a further group of proline-rich proteins, *Arch. Oral Biol.* **19**:627–632.

Hay, D. I., Smith, D. J., Schluckebier, S. K., and Moreno, E. C., 1984, Relationship between concentration of human salivary statherin and inhibition of calcium phosphate precipitation in stimulated human parotid saliva, *J. Dent. Res.* **63**:857–863.

Henkin, R. I., Lippoldt, R. E., Belstad, J., Wolf, R. O., Lum, C. K. L., and Edelhoch, H., 1978, Fractionation of human parotid saliva proteins, *J. Biol. Chem.* **253**:7556–7565.

Holbrook, I. B., and Molan, P. C., 1975, The identification of a peptide in human parotid saliva particularly active in enhancing the glycolytic activity of the salivary microorganisms, *Biochem. J.* **149**:489–492.

Ikemoto, S., Minaguchi, K., Suzuki, K., and Tomita, K., 1977, New genetic marker in human parotid saliva (Pm), *Science* **197**:378–379.

Ikemoto, S., Minaguchi, K., Tomita, T., and Suzuki, K., 1979, A variant protein in human parotid saliva detected by SDS polyacrylamide gel electrophoresis and its inheritance, *Ann. Hum. Genet.* **43**:11–14.

Ikemoto, S., Hinohara, H., Tsuchida, S., and Tomita, K., 1985, Phenotype and gene frequencies of acid phosphatase (s-AcP) in the human parotid saliva, *Hum. Genet.* **71**:30–32.

Ikemoto, S., Tsuchida, S., Hinohara, H., Nishiumi, E., Kajii, E., Nagai, K., Tomita, A., and Huang, D. Y., 1987, Further evidence for phenotypes and gene frequencies of nine salivary polymorphisms in Japanese population, *Forensic Sci. Int.* **35**:119–123.

Isemura, S., Saitoh, E., and Sanada, K., 1980, The amino acid sequence of a salivary proline-rich peptide, P-C, and its relation to a salivary proline-rich phosphoprotein, protein C, *J. Biochem.* **87**:1071–1077.

Isemura, S., Saitoh, E., and Sanada, K., 1982, Fractionation and characterization of basic proline-rich peptides of human parotid saliva and the amino acid sequence of proline-rich peptide P-E, *J. Biochem.* **91**:2067–2075.

Isemura, S., Saitoh, E., and Sanada, K., 1984, Isolation and amino acid sequence of SAP-1, an acidic protein of human whole saliva, and sequence homology with human γ-trace, *J. Biochem.* **96**:489–498.

Isemura, S., Saitoh, E., and Sanada, K., 1986a, Characterization of a new cysteine proteinase inhibitor of human saliva, cystatin SN, which is immunologically related to cystatin S, *FEBS Lett.* **198**:145–149.

Isemura, S., Saitoh, E., Sanada, K., Isemura, M., and Ito, S., 1986b, Cystatin S and the related cysteine proteinase inhibitors in human saliva, in: *Cysteine Proteinases and Their Inhibitors* (V. Turk, ed.), pp. 497–505, de Gruyter, Berlin.

Isemura, S., Saitoh, E., Sanada, K., Isemura, M., and Ito, S., 1986c, Cysteine proteinases of human saliva, *Acta Neurol. Scand.* **73**:317.

Ishizaki, K., Noda, A., Ikenaga, M., Omoto, K., Nakamura, Y., and Matsubara, K., 1985, Restriction fragment length polymorphism detected by human salivary amylase cDNA, *Hum. Genet.* **71**:261–262.

Ito, S., Suzuki, T., Momotsu, T., Isemura, S., Saitoh, E., Sanada, K., and Shibata, A., 1985, Presence of salivary protein C and salivary peptide P-C-like immunoreactivity in the laryngo-tracheo-bronchial glands, *Acta Endocrinol.* **108**:130–134.

Kamarýt, J., and Laxová, R., 1966, Amylase heterogeneity variants in man, *Humangenetik* **3**:41–45.

Karn, R. C., Friedman, R. D., and Merritt, A. D., 1979, Human salivary proline-rich (Pr) proteins: A post translational derivation of the phenotypes, *Biochem. Genet.* **17**:1061–1077.

Karn, R. C., Goodman, P. A., and Yu, P. L., 1985, Description of a genetic polymorphism of a human proline-rich salivary protein, Pc, and its relationship to other proteins in the salivary protein complex (SPC), *Biochem. Genet.* **23**:37–51.

Kauffman, D. L., and Keller, P. J., 1979, The basic-proline-rich proteins in human parotid saliva from a single subject, *Arch. Oral Biol.* **24**:249–256.

Kauffman, D., Wong, R., Bennick, A., and Keller, P., 1982, Basic proline-rich proteins from human parotid saliva: Complete covalent structure of protein IB-9 and partial structure of protein IB-6, members of a polymorphic pair, *Biochemistry* **21**:6558–6562.

Kauffman, D., Hofmann, T., Bennick, A., and Keller, P., 1986, Basic proline-rich proteins from parotid saliva: Complete covalent structures of proteins IB-I and IB-6, *Biochemistry* **25**:2387–2392.

Kim, H.-S., and Maeda, N., 1986, Structure of two *Hae*III-type genes in the human salivary proline-rich protein multigene family, *J. Biol. Chem.* **261**:6712–6718.

Kitamura, N., Kitagawa, H., Fukushima, D., Takagaki, Y., Takashi, M., and Nakanishi, S., 1985, Structural organization of the human kininogen gene and a model for its evolution, *J. Biol. Chem.* **260**:8610–8617.

Kühnl, P., and Tischberger, H., 1980, Amylase, polymorphism of human parotid saliva: Detection of a new allele Amy^5 by isoelectric focusing and Amy_1 population data from Germany, *Electrophoresis* **1**:186–190.

Levine, M. J., Weill, J. C., and Ellison, S. A., 1969, The isolation and analysis of a glycoprotein from parotid saliva, *Biochim. Biophys. Acta* **188**:165–167.

Lyons, K. M., Stein, J. H., and Smithies, O., 1988*a*, Length polymorphisms in human proline-rich protein genes generated by intragenic unequal crossing over, *Genetics* (in press).

Lyons, K. M., Azen, E. A., Goodman, P. A., and Smithies, O., 1988*b*, Many protein products from a few loci: Assignment of human salivary proline-rich proteins to specific loci, *Genetics* (in press).

Lyons, K. M., Kim H. S., Saitoh, E., and Smithies, O., submitted, Nucleotide sequences and evolution of the PRB3 and PRB4 genes from the human proline-rich protein multigene family (manuscript submitted).

MacKay, B. J., Pollock, J. J., Iacono, V. J., and Baum, B. J., 1984*a*, Isolation of milligram quantities of a group of histidine-rich polypeptides from human parotid saliva, *Infect. Immun.* **44**:688–694.

MacKay, B. J., Denepitiya, L., Iacono, V. J., Krost, S. B., and Pollock, J. J., 1984*b*, Growth-inhibitory and bactericidal effects of human parotid salivary histidine-rich polypeptides on *Streptococcus mutans, Infect. Immun.* **44**:695–701.

Maeda, N., 1985, Inheritance of human salivary proline-rich proteins: A reinterpretation in terms of six loci forming two subfamilies, *Biochem. Genet.* **23**:455–464.

Maeda, N., Kim, H.-S., Azen, E. A., and Smithies, O., 1985, Differential RNA splicing and post translational cleavages in the proline-rich protein gene system, *J. Biol. Chem.* **260**:11123–11130.

Mamula, P. W., Heerema, N. A., Palmer, C. G., Lyons, K. M., and Karn, R. C., 1985, Localization of the human salivary proteins complex (SPC) to chromosome band −12p13.2, *Cytogenet. Cell Genet.* **39**:279–284.

Mandel, I. D., and Bennick, A., 1983, Quantitation of human salivary acidic proline-rich proteins in oral disease, *J. Dent. Res.* **62**:943–945.

Mason, D. K., and Chisholm, D. M., 1975, Salivary glands and their secretions, in: *Salivary Glands in Health and Disease* (D. K. Mason and D. M. Chisholm, eds.), pp. 3–37, Saunders, London.

McKusick, V., 1986, *Mendelian Inheritance in Man. Categories of Autosomal Dominant, Autosomal Recessive, and X-Linked Phenotypes,* 7th ed., Johns Hopkins University Press, Baltimore, Maryland.

Mehansho, H., Hagerman, A., Clements, S., Butler, L., Rogler, J., and Carlson, D. M., 1983, Modulation of proline-rich protein biosynthesis in rat parotid glands by sorghums with high tannin levels, *Proc. Natl. Acad. Sci. USA* **80**:3948–3952.

Mehansho, H., Clements, S., Sheares, B. T., Smith, S., and Carlson, D. M., 1985, Induction of proline-rich glycoprotein synthesis in mouse salivary glands by isoproterenol and by tannins, *J. Biol. Chem.* **260**:4418–4423.

Mahansho, H., Butler, L. G., and Carlson, D. M., 1987, Dietary tannins and salivary proline-rich proteins: Interactions, induction and defense mechanisms, in: *Annual Review of Nutrition,* Vol. 7 (R. E. Olson, E. Beutler, and H. P. Broquist, eds.), pp. 423–440, Annual Reviews, Palo Alto, California.

Meisler, M., and Gumucio, D., 1986, Salivary amylase: Evolution and tissue-specific expression; and Pancreatic amylase: Molecular genetics and evolution, in: *Molecular and Cellular Basis of Digestion* (P. Desnuelle, H. Sjöström, and O. Norén, eds.), pp. 249–263 and 459–466, Elsevier, Amsterdam.

Merritt, A. D., and Karn, R. C., 1977, Human α-amylases, in: *Advances in Human Genetics,* Vol. 8 (H. Harris and K. Hirschhorn, eds.), pp. 135–234, Plenum Press, New York.

Minaguchi, K., and Suzuki, K., 1981, Frequencies of salivary genetic marker systems in Caucasians with an emphasis on Pm and Ph systems, *Forensic Sci. Int.* **17**:5–7.

Minaguchi, K., Ikemoto, S., and Suzuki, K., 1981*a*, Isolation and partial characterization of a polymorphic protein (Pm) in human parotid saliva, *Biochem. Genet.* **19**:617–621.

Minaguchi, K., Takaesu, Y., Tsutsumi, T., and Suzuki, K., 1981*b*, Studies of genetic markers in human saliva (VII) frequencies of the major parotid salivary glycoprotein (G1) system in a Japanese population, *Bull. Tokyo Dent. Coll.* **22**:1–6.

Minaguchi, K., Shirotani, T., and Suzuki, K., 1988, New variants of Ps salivary polymorphic proteins, *Ann. Hum. Genet.* **52**:11–16.

Minakato, K., and Asano, M., 1984, New protein inhibitors of cysteine proteinases in human saliva and salivary glands, *Hoppe-Seyler's Z. Physiol. Chem.* **365**:399–403.

Muenzer, J., Bildstein, C., Gleason, M., and Carlson, D. M., 1979, Purification of proline-rich proteins from parotid glands of isoproterenol-treated rats, *J. Biol. Chem.* **254**:5623–5628.

Müller-Esterl, W., Fritz, H., Kellerman, J., Lottopeich, F., Machleidt, W., and Turk, V., 1986, The mammalian cysteine proteinase inhibitors. Structural diversity and evolutionary origin, in: *Cysteine Proteinases and Their Inhibitors* (V. Turk, ed.), pp. 369–392, de Gruyter, Berlin.

Nakamura, Y., Ogawa, M., Nishide, T., Emi, M., Kosaki, G., Himeno, S., and Matsubara, K., 1984, Sequences of cDNA for human salivary and pancreatic α-amylases, *Gene* **28**:263–270.

Nishide, T., Emi, M., Nakamura, Y., and Matsubara, K., 1986*a*, Corrected sequences of cDNAs for human salivary and pancreatic α-amylases, *Gene* **50**:371–372.

Nishide, T., Nakamura, Y., Emi, M., Yamamoto, T., Ogawa, M., Mori, T., and Matsubara, K., 1986*b*, Primary structure of human salivary α-amylase gene, *Gene* **41**:299–304.

Noraini, I., Tan, S. G., Gan, Y. Y., and Teng, Y. S., 1980, Salivary peroxidase, Pm and Ph protein polymorphisms in Malaysians, *Hum. Genet.* **56**:205–207.

O'Connell, P. O., Lathrop, G. M., Law, M., Leppert, M., Nakamura, Y., Hoff, M., Kumlin, E., Thomas, W., Elsner, T., Ballard, L., Goodman, P., Azen, E., Sadler, J. E., Cai, G. Y., Lalovel, J. M., and White, R., 1987, A primary linkage map for human chromosome 12, *Genomics* **1**:93–102.

Oppenheim, F. G., Hay, D. I., and Franzblau, C., 1971, Proline-rich proteins from human parotid saliva. I. Isolation and partial characterization, *Biochemistry* **10**:4233–4238.

Oppenheim, F. G., Yang, Y. C., Diamond, R. D., Hyslop, D., Offner, G. D., and Troxler, R. F., 1986, The primary structure and functional characterization of the neutral histidine-rich polypeptide from human parotid secretion, *J. Biol. Chem.* **261**:1177–1182.

Peters, E. H., and Azen, E. A., 1977, Isolation and partial characterization of human parotid basic proteins, *Biochem. Genet.* **15**:925–946.

Peters, E. H., Goodfriend, T., and Azen, E. A., 1977, Human Pb, human post-Pb and non human primate Pb proteins: Immunological and biochemical relationships, *Biochem. Genet.* **15**:947–962.

Pollock, J. J., Denepitiya, L., MacKay, B. J., and Iacono, V., 1984, Fungistatic and fungicidal activity of human parotid salivary histidine-rich polypeptides on *Candida albicans*, *Infect. Immun.* **44**:702–707.

Pronk, J. C., 1977, A genetic variant of human salivary amylase detected by isoelectric focusing, in: *Electrofocusing and Isotachophoresis* (R. J. Radola and D. Graesslin, eds.), pp. 359–366, de Gruyter, Berlin.

Pronk, J. C., and Frants, R. R., 1979, New genetic variants of parotid salivary amylase, *Hum. Hered.* **29**:181–186.

Pronk, J. C., Frants, R. R., Jansen, W., Ericksson, A. W., and Tonino, G. J. M., 1982, Evidence for duplication of the human salivary amylase gene, *Hum. Genet.* **60**:32–35.

Pronk, J. C., Jansen, W. M., Pronk, A., Christian, F. A. M., Frants, R. R., and Erickson, A. W., 1984, Salivary protein polymorphism in Kenya: Evidence for a new Amy 1 allele, *Hum. Hered.* **34**:212–286.

Sabatini, L. M., Carlock, L. R., Johnson, G. W., and Azen, E. A., 1987, cDNA cloning and chromosomal localization of a gene (4q11–13) for statherin, a regulator of calcium in saliva, *Am. J. Hum. Genet.* **41**:1048–1060.

Saitoh, E., Isemura, S., and Sanada, K., 1983*a*, Complete amino acid sequence of a basic proline-rich peptide P-F, from human parotid saliva, *J. Biochem.* **93**:883–888.

Saitoh, E., Isemura, S., and Sanada, K., 1983*b*, Further fractionation of basic proline-rich peptides from human parotid saliva and complete amino acid sequence of basic proline-rich peptide P-H, *J. Biochem.* **94:**1991–1999.

Saitoh, E., Isemura, S., and Sanada, K., 1983*c*, Complete amino acid sequence of a basic proline-rich peptide, P-D, from human parotid saliva, *J. Biochem.* **93:**495–502.

Saitoh, E., Kim, H.-S., Smithies, O., and Maeda, N., 1987, Human cysteine-proteinase inhibitors: Nucleotide sequence analysis of three members of the cystatin gene family, *Gene* **61:**329–338.

Salvesen, G., Parkes, C., Rawlings, N. D., Brown, M. A., and Barrett, A. J., 1986, Cystatin-like domains of LMW-kininogens, and speculations on the origins of cystatins, in: *Cysteine Proteinases and Their Inhibitors* (V. Turk, ed.), pp. 413–428, de Gruyter, Berlin.

Schlesinger, D. H., and Hay, D. I., 1977, The complete covalent structure of statherin, a tyrosine-rich acidic peptide which inhibits calcium phosphate precipitation from human parotid saliva, *J. Biol. Chem.* **252:**1689–1695.

Shimomura, H., Kanai, Y., and Sanada, K., 1983, Amino acid sequences of glycopeptides obtained from basic proline-rich glycoprotein of human parotid saliva, *J. Biochem.* **93:**857–863.

Sung, M., and Smithies, O., 1969, Differential elution of histones from gel-trapped nuclei, *Biopolymers* **7:**39–58.

Tan, S. G., 1976, Human salivary esterases: Genetic studies, *Hum. Hered.* **26:**207–216.

Tan, S. G., and Ashton, G. C., 1976*a*, An autosomal glucose-6-phosphate dehydrogenase (hexose-6-phosphate dehydrogenase) polymorphism in human saliva, *Hum. Hered.* **26:**113–123.

Tan, S. G., and Ashton, G. C., 1976*b*, Saliva acid phosphatases: Genetic studies, *Hum. Hered.* **26:**81–89.

Tan, S. G., and Teng, Y. S., 1979, Human saliva as a source of genetic markers. I. Techniques, *Hum. Hered.* **29:**69–76.

Teng, Y. S., and Tan, S. G., 1979, Human saliva as a source of genetic markers. II. Genetic interpretations and possible utilizations, *Hum. Hered.* **29:**129–133.

Tenovuo, J., and Pruitt, K. M., 1984, Relationship of the human salivary peroxidase system to oral health, *J. Oral Pathol.* **13:**573–584.

Tricoli, J. V., and Shows, T. B., 1984, Regional assignment of human amylase (AMY) to p22 → p21 of chromosome 1, *Somat. Cell. Mol. Genet.* **10:**205–210.

Vining, R. F., and McGinley, R. A., 1986, Hormones in saliva, in: *CRC Critical Reviews in Clinical Laboratory Sciences,* Vol. 23 (J. Batsakis and J. Savory, eds.), pp. 95–146, CRC Press, Boca Raton, Florida.

Warner, T. F., and Azen, E. A., 1984, Proline-rich proteins are present in serous cells of the submucosal glands of the respiratory tract, *Am. Rev. Respir. Dis.* **130:**115–118.

Warner, T. F., and Azen, E. A., 1988, Tannins, salivary proline-rich proteins and esophageal cancer, *Med. Hypotheses* **26**(2).

Warner, T. F., Seo, I. S., Azen, E. A., Hafez, G. R., and Zarling, T. A., 1985, Immunocytochemistry of acinic carcinomas and mixed tumors of salivary glands, *Cancer* **56:**2221–2227.

Wise, R. J., Karn, R. C., Larsen, S. H., Hodes, M. E., Gardell, S. J., and Rutter,

W. J., 1984, A complementary DNA sequence that predicts a human pancreatic amylase primary structure consistent with the electrophoretic mobility of the common isozyme, Amy$_2$A, *Mol. Biol. Med.* **2**:307–322.

Wong, R. S. C., and Bennick, A., 1980, The primary structure of a salivary calcium-binding proline-rich phosphoprotein (protein C), a possible precursor of a related salivary protein A, *J. Biol. Chem.* **255**:5943–5948.

Wong, R. S. C., Hoffmann, T., and Bennick, A., 1979, The complete primary structure of a proline-rich phosphoprotein from human saliva, *J. Biol. Chem.* **254**:4800–4808.

Wong, R. S. C., Madapallimattam, G., and Bennick, A., 1983, The role of glandular kallikrein in the formation of a salivary proline-rich protein by cleavage of a single bond in salivary protein C, *Biochem. J.* **211**:35–44.

Yang, S. Y., Coleman, P. S., and Dupont, B., 1982, The biochemical and genetic basis for the microheterogeneity of human R-type vitamin B$_{12}$ binding proteins, *Blood* **59**:747–755.

Young, R. A., Hagenbuchle, O., and Schibler, U., 1981, A single mouse amylase gene specifies two different tissue-specific RNAs, *Cell* **23**:451–458.

Yu, P.-L., Karn, R. C., Merritt, A. D., Azen, E. A., and Conneally, P. M., 1980, Linkage relationships and multipoint mapping of the human parotid salivary proteins (Pr, Pa, Db), *Am. J. Hum. Genet.* **32**:555–563.

Yu, P.-L., Bixler, D., Goodman, P. A., Azen, E. A., and Karn, R. C., 1986, Human parotid proline-rich proteins: Correlation of genetic polymorphisms to dental caries, *Genet. Epidemiol.* **3**:147–152.

Zabel, B. U., Naylor, S. L., Sakaguchi, A. Y., Bell, G. I., and Shows, T. B., 1983, High-resolution chromosomal localization of human genes for amylase proopiomelanocortin, somatostatin, and a DNA fragment (D3S1) by *in situ* hybridization, *Proc. Natl. Acad. Sci. USA* **80**:6932–6936.

Ziemer, M. A., Mason, A., and Carlson, D. M., 1982, Cell free translations of proline-rich protein mRNAs, *J. Biol. Chem.* **256**:11176–11180.

Ziemer, M. A., Swain, W. F., Rutter, W. J., Clements, S., Ann, D. K., and Carlson, D. M., 1984, Nucleotide sequence analysis of a proline-rich protein cDNA and peptide homologies of rat and human proline-rich proteins, *J. Biol. Chem.* **259**:10475–10480.

Addendum

CHAPTER 2: THE MOLECULAR GENETICS OF HEMOPHILIA A AND B IN MAN
Factor VIII and Factor IX Deficiency

Stylianos E. Antonarakis

A number of additional mutations have been described in the factor VIII and factor IX gene since the submission of this chapter. Some deletions and point mutations will not be described here because their nature is the same as those described in the chapter. However, a novel mechanism of mutations in man has recently been discovered in the factor VIII gene (Kazazian *et al.*, 1988), namely *de novo* insertions of LINE repetitive elements into its coding regions.

L1 sequences are a human-specific family of long, interspersed, repetitive elements present in about 10^5 copies dispersed throughout the genome. The full length L1 sequence is 6.1 kb, but the majority of L1 elements are truncated at the 5' end, resulting in a fivefold higher copy number of 3' sequences (Skowronski and Singer, 1986). The nucleotide sequence of L1 elements includes an A-rich 3' end and two long open reading frames (ORF-1 and ORF-2), the second of which encodes a potential polypeptide with homology to reverse transcriptases (Skowronski and Singer, 1986). This structure suggests that L1 elements represent a class of non-viral retrotransposons (Scott *et al.*, 1987). A number of L1 cDNAs, including a nearly

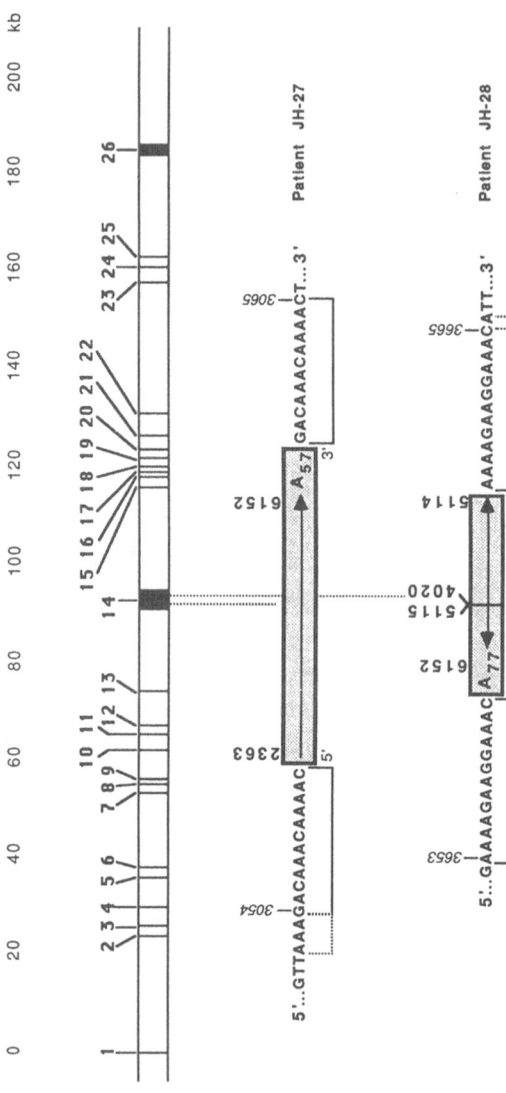

Fig. 11. Diagram of L1 insertions in exon 14 of the factor VIII gene. The 3.8-kb L1 insertion from patient JH-27 is flanked by a 12-bp target-site duplication of factor VIII cDNA sequence (nucleotides 3054–3065, where nucleotide 1 is the A of the initiator codon). Residues 3051–3053 of the factor VIII cDNA are adenylic acids and could also be duplicated (shown by the hatched bracket). The rearranged 2.3-kb insertion from patient JH-28 is shown and is flanked by a 13-bp target-site duplication. Residue 3666 of the factor VIII cDNA is an A and could be duplicated. Filled boxes represent the L1 elements, and the arrows within the boxes point toward the 3′ end of the L1 sequence. Both L1 insertions showed 98% similarity to the consensus genomic L1 sequence outside of the 3′ trailer region.

full-length element, have been isolated from an undifferentiated teratocarcinoma cell line (Skowronski and Singer, 1986). We have found insertions of L1 elements into exon 14 of the factor VIII gene in two of 240 unrelated patients with hemopilia A (Kazazian *et al.*, 1987). In both cases the parent did not have the insertion and, therefore, the event occurred *de novo*. Both of these insertions (3.8 kb and 2.3 kb) contained 3' portions of the L1 sequence, including the poly A tract, and created target site duplications of at least 12 and 13 nucleotides of the factor VIII gene (Fig. 11). In addition, their 3' trailer sequences following ORF-2 are nearly identical to the consensus sequence of L1 cDNAs. The data indicate that in man certain L1 sequences can be dispersed, presumably via an RNA intermediate, and cause disease by insertional mutation.

Insertion of L1 elements, involving retrotransposition of DNA sequences through an RNA intermediate into a new and distant location in the genome, represents a fundamentally different mechanism of mutation-producing human disease from those previously described. Because we do not know when these L1-insertions events occur—whether in the sperm or ovum, after fertilization, or during early stages of embryogenesis—the proportion of such insertions that are heritable is unknown. Finding two L1 insertions among 240 patients with hemophilia A, however, suggests that this mechanism of mutation is not uncommon.

REFERENCES

Kazazian, H. H., Jr., Wong, C., Youssoufian, H., Scott, A. F., Phillips, D. G., and Antonarakis, S. E., 1987, A novel mechanism of mutation in man: Hemophilia due to *de novo* insertion of L1 sequences, *Nature* **332**:165–166.

Scott, A. F., Schmeckpeper, B. J., Abdelrazik, M., Theisen Comey, C., O'Hara, B., Pratt Rossiter, J., Cooley, T., Heath, P., Smith, K. D., and Margolet, L., 1987, Origin of the human L1 elements: Proposed progenitor genes deduced from a consensus DNA sequences, *Genomics* **1**:113–125.

Skowronski, J., and Singer, M. F., 1986, The abundant LINE-1 family of repeated DNA sequences in mammals: Genes and pseudogenes, *Cold Spring Harbor Symp. Quant. Biol.* **51**:457–464.

Index

Abortion, spontaneous
  and imbalance, chromosomal, 99
Acetic acid, 8
Acid phosphatase, salivary, 151,
    152, 156
Adrenoleukodystrophy, 53
Age, maternal
  and heteromorphism,
      cytogenetic, 103
  hypothesis of
    older egg, 102
    relaxed selection, 103
  and polymorphism of DNA, 103
  and trisomy 21, 102–104
Aldolase, 63
Amniocentesis, 1
Amylase, salivary, 143
  gene family, 187–189
  variant, genetic, 154
Aneuploidy, 10
Aspiration technique
  transabdominal, 7–8
  transcervical, 4–6

B$_{12}$-binding protein, salivary, 150,
    151, 155
  gastric intrinsic factor, 155
  polymorphism, 155
  R-protein, 155
  sources, 155
  transcobalamin II, 155

Becker muscular dystrophy, 62–98
  gene deletion, 71–79
  laboratory findings, 63
  muscle-wasting disorder, 62
  "outliers," 62
  protein, 87–89
  translocation X:autosome, 66
  X-linked trait, recessive, 62
Biopsy forceps, 4–7
  guided by
    endoscope, 4
    ultrasound, 4, 6
  transcervical, 6–7

Calcium, 156, 185
  homeostasis, 64
  metabolism, 64
Catheter aspiration, transcervical,
    4–6
Centromere mapping, 130–131
Chiasma frequency, 107
Christmas disease: see Hemophilia
    B
Chromosome
  acrocentric, exchange of, 111
  walking, 74, 78, 113, 115
  21: see Trisomy 21
    crossing-over, 106–109
      and nondisjunction, 106–109
    DNA probes, polymorphic,
        single-copy
      on long arm, 118–122

Chromosome (*cont.*)
21 (*cont.*)
    DNA sequences, 110–112
    imbalance and disorder,
        congenital, 99
    organization, cytogenetic,
        110–126
    DNA sequences, 110–112
    long arm and DNA probes,
        118–122
    short arm, acrocentric,
        110–118
    organization of the region,
        pericentromeric, 118
Clotting factor deficiency: *see*
    Hemophilia
Color blindness, 53
Couples at high risk for trisomy 21,
    104–106
    factors listed
        extrinsic, 104
        intrinsic, 104
Creatine phosphokinase, 63
Cystatin, salivary, gene family,
    189–191
Cysteine-proteinase inhibitor: *see*
    Cystatin

Delta lesion, 63
Diagnosis of defect, genetic, 1–25;
        see also Villus, chorionic
DNA
    analysis of villus, chorionic, 4,
        15–16
    polymorphism
        and nondisjunction, 120–121
        and recombination, 121–122
    sequence on chromosome, short-
        arm, acrocentric, 110–112
    Southern blot hybridization, 176
Down syndrome: *see* Trisomy 21

Duchenne muscular dystrophy,
    61–98
aspect
    biochemical, 63–65
    clinical, 62–63
calcium homeostasis, 64
chromsome map position of the
    locus of, 65–67, 81–87, 89
death, 62
deletions, 66–67, 70–79
delta lesion, 63
DNA
    cloned, 67–71, 76, 79
    recombination, 69–70
exons, 79–80, 84–86
genes
    cloned, 61
    identified, 61
    locus, 65–67, 81–87, 89
        schema of, 83
    strategy approach to, 67–71
    transcript, identification of,
        79–81
introns, 79
laboratory findings, 63
muscle weakness is progressive,
    62
membrane theory of etiology,
    63, 65
penetrance, 62
protein, 87–89
and retardation, mental, 87
X-linked trait, recessive, 62
Dystrophy, muscular: *see* Becker,
    Duchenne

Endometrium, 2
Endoscopy, transcervical, 6

Fibrin, 27
Forceps for biopsy, transcervical,
    6–7